● ● ● ● ● ● ● ● ● ● ● ● ●

Jennifer grun

POCKET
PSYCH
DRUGS

Point-of-Care Clinical Guide

Darlene D. Pedersen, MSN, APRN,
PMHCNS, BC

In consultation with
Laura G. Leahy, MSN, APN, CNS, FNP, BC

Purchase additional copies of this book at your health science
bookstore or directly from F.A. Davis by shopping online
at www.fadavis~ ~ ~ ~ ~alling 800-3?? ?0?? ~ ~r
800-665-1148

F. A. Davis Company
1915 Arch Street
Philadelphia, PA 19103
www.fadavis.com

Printed in China by Imago

Last digit indicates print number: 10 9 8 7 6 5 4 3 2 1

Publisher, Nursing: Robert G. Martone
Senior Developmental Editor: William F. Welsh
Senior Project Editor: Padraic J. Maroney
Manager of Art & Design: Carolyn O'Brien
Reviewers: Lois Angelo, APRN, MSN, Laura Aromando, ARNP, MSN, Barbara Braverman, MSN, CRNP, BC-
CNS, Arleen F. Briggs, RN, MSN, FNC, ARNP, Barbara Chamberlain, PhD, APRN, CCRN, WCC, Perri-Anne
Concialdi, RN, MSN, CNS, Karen I. Curtis, PMHCNS-BC, Margie Eckroth-Bucher, PhD, RN, PMHCNS-BC,
Kathryn Farwell, PhD, RN, Elizabeth A. Favreau, MSN, RN, CNE, Linda S. Forte, Carlile Frederick, APRN,
PMH-BC, CRNP, Melissa Garno, EdD, Sheila Hart, MSN, RN, Joan Hoover, RN, BSN, MSEd, Dottie Irvin,
DNS, APRN, BC, Florence Keane, DNSc, MBA, ARNP-FNP-C, Michelle Link, RN, MSN, Angela Luciani, RN,
BScN, MN, Robin Murray, RN, MSN, Ketankumar V. Patel, MD, Catherine Ann Weitzel, RN, MSN, ARNP

As new scientific information becomes available through basic and clinical research, recommended
treatments and drug therapies undergo changes. The author(s) and publisher have done everything
possible to make this book accurate, up to date, and in accord with accepted standards at the time of
publication. The author(s), editors, and publisher are not responsible for errors or omissions or for conse-
quences from application of the book, and make no warranty, expressed or implied, in regard to the contents of the book. Any practice described in this book should be applied by the reader in accordance
with professional standards of care used in regard to the unique circumstances that may apply in each
situation. The reader is advised always to check product information (package inserts) for changes and
new information regarding dose and contraindications before administering any drug. Caution is especially urged when using new or infrequently ordered drugs.

Contents

● ● ● ● ● ● ● ● ● ● ● ●

The following resources can be found on DavisPlus (http://davisplus.fadavis.com):
– Algorithms in Psychopharmacology [Generalized Anxiety Disorder, Post-Traumatic Stress Disorder, and Schizophrenia; Spanish: Generalized Anxiety Disorder and Post-Traumatic Stress Disorder] © Copyright 2004-2006. International Psychopharmacology Algorithm Project (IPAP) www.ipap.org [see General Resources]
– Animations [Anxiety Disorders, Depression, Schizophrenia, Pharmacokinetics: ADME] [see General and Student Resources]
– Client Education Teaching Guides (Client/Family Handouts)[see General and Student Resources]
– Davis's Dosage Calculator [see General and Student Resources]
– Laboratory Medication Levels [Anticonvulsant Drugs, Antidepressants, Antipsychotic Drugs and Antimanics] [see General and Student Resources]
– Medication Assessment Tool [see General and Student Resources]
– Preventing Medication Errors [see General and Student Resources]
– Psychotropic Drug Monographs [see General and Student Resources]
– Psychotropic Medication Tutorial [see General and Student Resources]
– Syringe Compatibility Chart [see General and Student Resources]
– Syringe Exercises [see General and Student Resources]

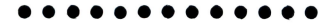

Basics of Psychopharmacology/Biology and Drug Classes

Pharmacokinetics/Pharmacodynamics

Pharmacokinetics (PK) can be defined as "how the body processes a drug" resulting in a drug's concentration in the body. This is done through absorption, distribution, metabolism, and excretion (ADME).

Absorption: Describes the drug's movement from point of administration (oral, injection, skin) until it reaches the bloodstream. In oral administration, **first-pass metabolism** refers to how much of the drug is metabolized by the liver and therefore is not available to the bloodstream (bioavailability of drug). This determines the dose needed for oral administration or the need for an alternative route of entry (such as parenteral).

Distribution: Movement of drug from the bloodstream to the rest of the body. Concerned with movement over the blood-brain barrier (may affect the brain) or crossing the placenta (may affect the fetus). Also concerns highly protein-bound drugs that may cause drug interactions.

Metabolism and Excretion: The primary organ of metabolism is the liver, and excretion of drugs takes place through the kidneys. Dosing considerations are based on how well the liver and kidneys are functioning. Half-life is also a factor as drugs with long half-lives may accumulate, resulting in overdose or toxicity.

Half-life is the time (hours) that it takes for 50% of a drug to be eliminated from the body. Time to total elimination involves halving the remaining 50%, and so forth, until total elimination. Half-life is considered in determining dosing frequency and in determining time to steady state. The rule of thumb for **steady state** (stable concentration/manufacture effect) **attainment** is 4–5 half-lives. *Because of fluoxetine's long half-life, a 5-week washout is recommended after stopping fluoxetine and before starting an MAOI to avoid a serious and possibly fatal reaction.*

Protein Binding is the amount of drug that binds to the blood's plasma proteins; the remainder circulates unbound. It is important to understand this concept when prescribing two or more highly protein-bound drugs as one drug may be displaced, causing increased blood levels and adverse effects.

Pharmacodynamics is usually defined as "what the drug does to the body" and therefore the effect the drug has on the body (positive effects and side effects).

Cytochrome P-450 Enzyme System is involved in drug biotransformation and metabolism. It is important to develop a knowledge of this system to understand drug metabolism and especially drug interactions. Over 30 P-450 isoenzymes have been identified. The major isoenzymes include CYP1A2/2A6/2B6/2C8/2C9/2C18/2C19/2D6/2E1/3A4/3A5-7.

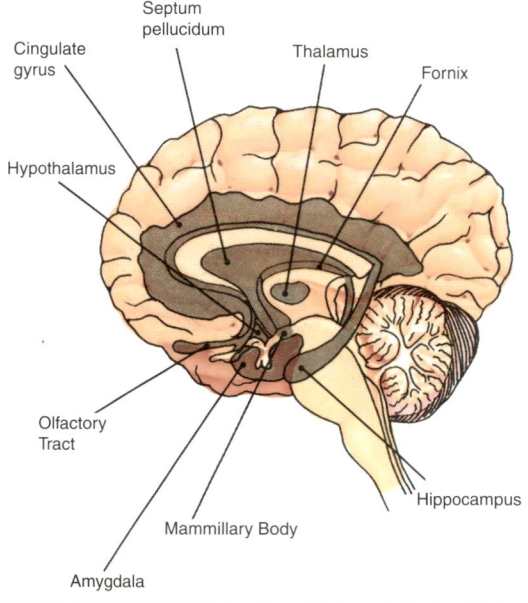

The limbic system and its structures (*Adapted from Scanlon VC, Sanders T: Essentials of Anatomy and Physiology, ed. 5. FA Davis, Philadelphia 2007, with permission*)

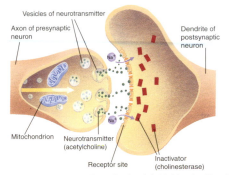

Impulse transmission at a synapse. Arrow indicates direction of electrical impulse. *(From Scanlon VC, Sanders T: Essentials of Anatomy and Physiology, ed. 5. FA Davis, Philadelphia 2007, with permission)*

Autonomic Nervous System

SYMPATHETIC AND PARASYMPATHETIC EFFECTS

Structure	Sympathetic	Parasympathetic
Eye (pupil)	Dilation	Constriction
Nasal mucosa	Mucus reduced	Mucus increased
Salivary gland	Saliva reduced	Saliva increased
Heart	Rate increased	Rate decreased
Arteries	Constriction	Dilation
Lung	Bronchial muscle relaxation	Bronchial muscle contraction
Gastrointestinal tract	Decreased motility	Increased motility
Liver	Conversion of glycogen to glucose increased	Glycogen synthesis
Kidney	Decreased urine	Increased urine
Bladder	Contraction of sphincter	Relaxation of sphincter
Sweat glands	↑ Sweating	No change

(From Pedersen: PsychNotes, 2e, 2008, with permission)

BASICS

NEUROTRANSMITTER FUNCTIONS AND EFFECTS

Neurotransmitter	Function	Effect
Dopamine	Inhibitory	Fine movement, emotional behavior; ↓ ↑ in schizophrenia and ↑ Parkinson's. Implicated in addiction.
Serotonin	Inhibitory	Sleep, mood, eating behavior. Implicated in mood disorders, anxiety, and violence.
Norepinephrine	Excitatory	Arousal, wakefulness, learning. Implicated in anxiety, ADHD, and "fight or flight reaction."
GABA	Inhibitory	Anxiety states.
Acetylcholine	Excitatory	Arousal, attention, movement. Increase = spasms and decrease = paralysis.

(From Pedersen: PsychNotes, 2e, 2008, with permission)

Medication and the Elderly

- Relevant drug guides provide data about dosing for the elderly and debilitated clients. (See also Drug/tabs.)
- Elderly and debilitated clients are started at lower doses, often half the recommended adult dose. This is due to:
  - Decreases in GI absorption
  - Decrease in total body water (decreased plasma volume)
  - Decreased lean muscle and increased adipose tissue
  - Reduced first-pass effect in the liver and cardiac output
  - Decreased serum albumin
  - Decreased glomerular filtration and renal tubular secretion
  - Time to steady state is prolonged

Because of decrease in lean muscle mass and increase in fat (retains lipophilic drugs [fat-storing]), reduced first-pass metabolism, and decreased renal function, drugs may remain in the body longer and produce an additive effect.

Clinical Tips/Alert: With the elderly, start doses low and titrate slowly. Drugs that result in postural hypotension, confusion, or sedation should be used cautiously or not at all.

- **Poor Drug Choices for the Elderly -** Drugs that cause postural hypotension or anticholinergic side effects (sedation).
  - *TCAs* - anticholinergic (confusion, constipation, visual blurring); cardiac (conduction delay; tachycardia); alpha-1 adrenergic (orthostatic hypotension [falls])
  - *Benzodiazepines*- longer the half-life, the greater the risk of falls. May also increase agitation and confusion. Choose a shorter half-life. Lorazepam (T $1/2$ 12 15 hr) is a better choice than diazepam (T $1/2$ 20-70 hr; metabolites up to 200 hr).
  - *Lithium* - use cautiously in elderly, especially if debilitated. Risk of dehydration may yield lithium toxicity.
  - *Diphenhydramine* (Benadryl; Canada: Allerdryl) – $\uparrow$ susceptibility to adverse reactions/anticholinergic effects (delirium, dizziness, confusion).
  - Consider age, weight, mental state, and medical disorders and compare with side-effect profile in selecting medications.

Pharmacokinetics in the Elderly

Pharmacokinetics is the way that a drug is absorbed, distributed and used, metabolized, and excreted by the body. Age-related physiological changes affect body systems, altering pharmacokinetics and increasing or altering a drug's effect.

x

Physiological Change		Effect on Pharmacokinetics
Absorption	• Decreased intestinal motility	• Delayed peak effect
	• Diminished blood flow to the gut	• Delayed signs/symptoms of toxic effects
Distribution	• Decreased body water	• Increased serum concentration of water-soluble drugs
	• Increased percentage of body fat	• Increased half-life of fat-soluble drugs
	• Decreased amount of plasma proteins	• Increased amount of active drug
Metabolism	• Decreased lean body mass	• Increased drug concentration
	• Decreased blood flow to liver	• Decreased rate of drug clearance by liver
	• Diminished liver function	• Increased accumulation of some drugs
Excretion	• Diminished kidney function	• Increased accumulation of some drugs
	• Decreased creatinine clearance	• Decreased drugs excreted by kidney

(From Myers, RNotes, 2e, 2006, p. 97, with permission)

Medications and Children

Indications/Off-Label Uses: The majority of psychotropic medications are used "off-label" in children. The exceptions to this are those with the following FDA-Approved Clinical Indications:

Attention-Deficit Hyperactivity Disorder (ADHD) Medications: amphetamine salts (ages ≥3), methylphenidate (ages ≥6), lisdexamfetamine (ages ≥6), atomoxetine (ages ≥6)

Selective Serotonin Reuptake Inhibitor (SSRI) Antidepressants: fluoxetine for depression (ages 8–18) and obsessive compulsive disorder (ages 7–18) and sertraline for obsessive compulsive disorder (ages 6–17)

Atypical Antipsychotic Medications: aripiprazole for adolescent schizophrenia (ages 3–17), bipolar mania (ages 10–17), adjunct treatment of bipolar mania (ages 10–17), and risperidone] irritability related to autistic disorder (ages 5–16)

Although the majority of psychotropic medications do not have an FDA-approved indication, there is significant research and data on most of these medications providing a base of evidence to guide the clinician in his/her decision making when prescribing for children and adolescents (Martin & Lewis 2006).

Pediatric Dosing: As with the elderly, when prescribing psychotropic medications for children and adolescents, it is prudent to start at subtherapeutic doses and titrate slowly to minimize any potential adverse events and/or side effects. Maximizing one medication before augmenting is also helpful when working with children and adolescents to avoid exacerbation of symptoms and side effects. Additionally, it is essential to review the side effects, risks, benefits, and alternatives with the client and caregiver, as the majority of psychotropics do not have FDA-approved indications for use in children and adolescents.

> **Clinical Tips/Alert:** Children generally do not like to take medications. If the child's symptoms warrant intervention with a psychotropic medication, it is essential to evaluate the potential for compliance. Fortunately, many of the psychotropic medications are available in liquid form or as capsules, which can be opened and whose contents are sprinkled on soft foods. Additionally, some medications have alternate delivery systems (e.g., fluoxetine weekly, methylphenidate transdermal, methylphenidate chewable, etc.), which may enhance adherence. *Convenience equals compliance, especially with children.*

Psychotropic Adverse Effects

Extrapyramidal Symptoms (EPS)

EPS are caused by antipsychotic treatment and need to be monitored/evaluated for early intervention.

- Akinesia – rigidity and bradykinesia.
- Akathisia – restlessness; movement of body; unable to keep still; movement of feet (do not confuse with anxiety).
- Dystonia – spasmodic and painful spasm of muscle (torticollis [head pulled to one side]).
- Oculogyric crisis – eyes roll back toward the head. **This is an emergency situation.**
- Pseudoparkinsonism – simulates Parkinson's disease with shuffling gait, drooling, muscular rigidity, and tremor.
- Rabbit syndrome – rapid movement of the lips that simulates a rabbit's mouth movements.

Tardive Dyskinesia

Permanent dysfunction of voluntary muscles. Affects the mouth - tongue protrudes, smacking of lips, mouth movements; also involves fingers and extremities.

[**Clinical Tips/Alert:** Evaluate client on antipsychotics for possible tardive dyskinesia by using the AIMS.]

Neuroleptic Malignant Syndrome (NMS)

A serious and potentially fatal syndrome caused by antipsychotics and other drugs that block dopamine receptors. Important not to allow client to become *dehydrated* (predisposing factor). More common in warm climates, in summer. Possible genetic predisposition.

Signs and Symptoms
- Fever – 103°–105°F or greater
- BP lability (hypertension or hypotension)
- Tachycardia (>130 bpm)
- Tachypnea (>25 rpm)
- Agitation (respiratory distress, tachycardia)
- Diaphoresis, pallor
- Muscle rigidity (arm/abdomen like a board)
- Change in mental status (stupor to coma)

Stop antipsychotic immediately

[**Clinical Tips/Alert:** NMS is a medical emergency (10% mortality rate); hospitalization needed. Lab test: Creatinine kinase (CK) to determine injury to the muscle. Drugs used to treat NMS include: bromocriptine, dantrolene, levodopa, lorazepam.]

Serotonin Syndrome

Can occur if client is taking one or more serotonergic drugs (e.g., SSRIs; St. John's wort), especially higher doses. Do not combine SSRIs/SNRIs/clomipramine with MAOIs; tryptophan or dextromethorphan combined with an MAOI can produce this syndrome. If stopping fluoxetine (long half-life) to start an MAOI – must allow a 5–week washout period. At least 2 weeks for other SSRIs before starting an MAOI. Discontinue the MAOI for 2 weeks before starting another antidepressant or other interacting drug.

Signs and Symptoms

- Change in mental status, agitation, confusion, restlessness, flushing
- Diaphoresis, diarrhea, lethargy, nausea, vomiting
- Myoclonus (muscle twitching or jerks), tremors
- Hyperthermia, tachycardia

If serotonergic medication is not discontinued, progresses to:

- Worsening myoclonus, hypertension, rigor
- Acidosis, respiratory failure, rhabdomyolysis

> **Clinical Tips/Alert:** Must discontinue serotonergic medication immediately. Emergency medical treatment and hospitalization needed to treat myoclonus, hypertension, and other symptoms.

Treatment-Emergent Diabetes

It has been found that atypical antipsychotic use is associated with an increased risk of hyperglycemia-related adverse events and the possibility of treatment-emergent diabetes. This is especially true of olanzapine, but all atypicals carry this risk, and caution should be used with conventionals as well. Hyperglycemia with associated ketoacidosis or hyperosmolar coma or death has been associated with olanzapine and other atypicals (Ahuja et al, 2008). (*See Body Mass Index/Metabolic Syndrome in Tools tab.*)

Antiparkinsonian Agents

These are *anticholinergics* used to treat drug-induced parkinsonism and EPS (caused by dopamine and ACh imbalance). These include:

- Benztropine (Cogentin)
- Biperiden (Akineton)
- Trihexyphenidyl (Artane)
- Others, including amantadine (dopaminergic) and diphenhydramine (antihistaminic)

Anticholinergic side effects include:

- Blurred vision, dry mouth, constipation
- Sedation, urinary retention, and tachycardia

> **Clinical Tips/Alert:** Use cautiously in the elderly and cardiac arrhythmias.

Drug-Herbal Interactions

Antidepressants should not be used concurrently with: St. John's wort or SAMe (serotonin syndrome and/or altered antidepressant metabolism).

Benzodiazepines/sedative/hypnotics should not be used concurrently with chamomile, skullcap, valerian, or kava. St. John's wort may reduce the effectiveness of benzodiazepines metabolized by CYP P450 3A4.

Conventional antipsychotics (haloperidol, chlorpromazine) that are sedating should not be used in conjunction with chamomile, skullcap, valerian, or kava. Carbamazepine, clozapine, and olanzapine should not be used concurrently with St. John's wort (altered drug metabolism/effectiveness).

Clinical Tips/Alert: Ask all clients specifically what, if any, herbal or over-the-counter (OTC) medications they are using to treat symptoms. Review all OTC and herbal drugs for possible interactions with prescribed medications.

Therapeutic Drug Classes

Antianxiety (Anxiolytic) Agents

Used in the treatment of generalized anxiety, OCD, panic disorder, post-traumatic stress disorder (PTSD), phobic disorders, insomnia, and others and includes:

- benzodiazepines (alprazolam, clonazepam, lorazepam, oxazepam)
- buspirone
- alpha-2 adrenergics (clonidine)
- antihistamines (hydroxyzine)
- beta blockers (propranolol)
- antidepressants (doxepin, tricyclics, escitalopram, SSRIs)
- hyponsedatives for insomnia, such as zolpidem, eszopiclone

Antidepressant Agents

Used in the treatment of depression (depressed), bipolar, OCD, anxiety, and others and includes:

- tricyclics (amitriptyline, desipramine, doxepin, imipramine)
- MAOIs (phenelzine, tranylcypromine)
- SSRIs (fluoxetine, paroxetine, sertraline)
- SNRIs (venlafaxine, duloxetine)
- others (aminoketone/triazolopyridine) (bupropion trazodone)

Mood-Stabilizing Agents

Used in the treatment of bipolar disorder (mania/depression), aggression, schizoaffective, and others and includes:

- lithium
- anticonvulsants (valproic acid, carbamazepine, lamotrigine, topiramate)
- conventional and atypical antipsychotics (chlorpromazine, haloperidol, risperidone, aripiprazole, etc.)

Antipsychotic (Neuroleptic) Agents

Used in the treatment of schizophrenia, psychotic episodes (depression/organic [dementia]/substance-induced), bipolar disorder, agitation, delusional disorder, and others and includes:

- **Conventional antipsychotics:**
  - phenothiazines (chlorpromazine, thioridazine)
  - butyrophenones (haloperidol)
  - thioxanthenes (thiothixene)
  - diphenylbutyl piperidines (pimozide)
  - dibenzoxazepine (loxapine)
  - dyhydroindolone (molindone)
- **Atypical antipsychotics:**
  - dibenzodiazepine (clozapine)
  - benzisoxazole (risperidone)
  - thienobenzodiazepine (olanzapine)
  - benzothiazolyl piperazine (ziprasidone)
  - dihydrocarbostyril (aripiprazole)

Although other agents (e.g., stimulants) may be used in the treatment of psychiatric disorders, the most common therapeutic classes and agents are listed above.

Side Effects Associated With Therapeutic Classes

Antihypertensives (clonidine, propranolol): Drowsiness, dizziness, hypotension, nausea, constipation, bradycardia

Antianxiety (alprazolam, diazepam, lorazepam, oxazepam): Dizziness, drowsiness, confusion, hangover, paradoxical excitation, ataxia, blurred vision, constipation, diarrhea, nausea, psychological and physical dependence, withdrawal

Anticonvulsants/mood stabilizers (valproic acid, carbamazepine, lamotrigine, topiramate, clonazepam): Drowsiness, dizziness, rash, blood dyscrasias; Carbamazepine: AGRANULOCYTOSIS, APLASTIC ANEMIA, STEVENS-JOHNSON SYNDROME; Divalproex: HEPATOTOXICITY, PANCREATITIS; Lamotrigine: ↑ rash, STEVENS-JOHNSON SYNDROME; Topiramate: ↑ SEIZURES, SUICIDE ATTEMPT

Antidepressants: Heterocyclics (mirtazapine, trazodone, bupropion): Dizziness, sedation, headache, dry mouth, tachycardia; Trazodone: PRIAPISM; Bupropion: SEIZURES

MAOIs (phenelzine, tranylcypromine): Dizziness, insomnia, orthostatic hypotension, arrhythmias, diarrhea, SEIZURES, HYPERTENSIVE CRISIS

SNRIs (venlafaxine, duloxetine): Dry mouth, constipation, dizziness, insomnia, headache, sexual dysfunction; Venlafaxine: ↑ hypertension, SEIZURES; Nefazodone: HEPATIC FAILURE; Duloxetine: SEIZURES

SSRIs (fluoxetine, paroxetine, sertraline, escitalopram): Insomnia, anxiety, nausea (esp. paroxetine), drowsiness, diarrhea, constipation, sexual dysfunction, serotonin syndrome (emergency if untreated).

Tricyclics (amitriptyline, imipramine, nortriptyline): Dry mouth, blurred vision, nausea, vomiting, drowsiness, constipation, ARRHYTHMIAS, tachycardia, hypotension, ↑ seizure threshold

Antipsychotics: Atypical (olanzapine, risperidone, quetiapine): EPS (lower than conventionals) [risperidone ↑ risk of EPS with ↑ dose], NEUROLEPTIC MALIGNANT SYNDROME, hyperglycemia (diabetes), weight gain (esp. olanzapine), tardive dyskinesia (TD) (lower than conventionals), sedation, agitation. ↓ **mortality in elderly with dementia-related psychosis**

Conventional (chlorpromazine, haloperidol, thioridazine): EPS, NEUROLEPTIC MALIGNANT SYNDROME, SEIZURES, TD, blurred vision, dry mouth, hyperprolactinemia (galactorrhea, amenorrhea), hypotension, sedation, weight gain, tachycardia, arrhythmic effects, photosensitivity, ↑ **mortality in elderly with dementia-related psychosis**

Mood stabilizer: Antimanic: Lithium: Weight gain, acne, psoriatic arthritis, dry mouth, thirst, polyuria, diarrhea, ECG changes, hypothyroidism, tremors, SEIZURES, ARRHYTHMIAS

Sedative/hypnotics (ramelteon, zaleplon, zolpidem): Somnolence, dizziness, nausea, fatigue, headache, complex sleep-related behaviors, severe allergic reactions, ANA-PHYLACTIC REACTIONS

Side effects in ALL CAPS = Life-threatening

Black Box Warnings

Black Box Warnings are FDA Warnings of Potential Serious or Life Threatening Adverse Events Related to the Medication. Following are lists of FDA warnings followed by medications associated with these warnings:

Increased Risk of Suicidality (suicidal thinking & behavior) in Children, Adolescents, and Young Adults

- Tri- & heterocyclic Antidepressants (amitriptyline, clomipramine, desipramine, doxepin, imipramine, nortriptyline, trazodone)
- MAOI Antidepressants (tranylcypromine, isocarboxazid, selegiline, phenelzine)
- SSRI Antidepressants (citalopram, escitalopram, paroxetine, fluoxetine, sertraline, fluvoxamine)
- Other Antidepressants (duloxetine, venlafaxine, desvenlafaxine, mirtazapine, nefazodone, bupropion, atomoxetine)
- Atypical Antipsychotics (quetiapine, aripiprazole, olanzapine/fluoxetine)

Increased Risk of Mortality in Elderly with Dementia Related Psychosis
- ALL Conventional & Atypical Antipsychotics
High Potential for Abuse and Dependence with Misuse
- Amphetamines & Amphetamine Salts
Misuse May Lead to Sudden Death/Serious CV Events
- Amphetamines & Amphetamine Salts
Life Threatening Hepatic Failure/Potential for Severe Liver Injury

- Nefazodone
- Atomoxetine (bolded, not Black Boxed)

Serious Dermatological Reaction including toxic epidermal necrolysis and Stevens-Johnson Syndrome
- Carbamazepine
Aplastic Anemia and Agranulocytosis

- Carbamazepine
- Clozapine

Orthostatic Hypotension, Seizures & Convulsions
- Clozapine
(*Source:* fda.gov/cder/index)
(Check the fda.gov Web site for changes to/additions to Black Box warnings.)

BASICS

Psychotropic Drugs A–C

Alprazolam

(al-**pray**-zoe-lam) Xanax, Xanax XR, *Apo-Alpraz, Novo-Alprazol, Nirvam, Nu-Alpraz*

Classification: *Therapeutic:* Antianxiety agents; *Pharmacological:* Benzodiazepines; *Schedule IV; Pregnancy Category D*

Indications: Treatment of GAD; panic disorder; anxiety associated with depression.

Off-Label Use: Premenstrual syndrome (PMS), insomnia, IBS, somatic symptoms associated with anxiety, Acute mania, acute psychosis adjunct.

Action: Acts at many levels in CNS to produce anxiolytic effect. May produce CNS depression. Effects may be mediated by GABA, an inhibitory neurotransmitter.

Pharmacokinetics: *Absorption:* Well absorbed (90%) from GI tract; absorption slower with extended-release tablets.

Distribution: Widely distributed, crosses blood-brain barrier; Probably crosses placenta and enters breast milk. Accumulation minimal.

Metabolism and Excretion: Metabolized by liver (CYP3A4 enzyme system) to an active compound that is subsequently rapidly metabolized.

$T\frac{1}{2}$: 12–15 hr (intermediate).

TIME/ACTION PROFILE (sedation)

Route	Onset	Peak	Duration
PO	1–2 hr	1–2 hr	Up to 24 hr

Contraindicated in: *Pregnancy and Lactation:* Use in pregnancy or lactation may cause CNS depression, flaccidity, feeding difficulties, and seizures in infant. Hypersensitivity; cross-sensitivity with other benzodiazepines may exist; pre-existing CNS depression; severe uncontrolled pain; angle-closure glaucoma, obstructive sleep apnea, pulmonary disease; concurrent itraconazole or ketoconazole.

Use Cautiously in: Renal impairment, hepatic dysfunction (↓ dose required); concurrent use with nefazodone, fluvoxamine, cimetidine, fluoxetine, hormonal contraceptives, propoxyphene, diltiazem, isoniazid, erythromycin, clarithromycin, grapefruit juice (↓ dose may be necessary); history of suicide attempt or alcohol/drug dependence, debilitated clients (↓ dose required). SSRI antidepressants may potentiate effect.

Adverse Reactions/Side Effects (CAPITALS indicate life-threatening; <u>underlines</u> indicate most frequent)
CNS: <u>Dizziness</u>, <u>drowsiness</u>, <u>lethargy</u>, confusion, hangover, headache, mental depression, paradoxical excitation. **EENT:** Blurred vision. **GI:** Constipation, diarrhea, nausea, vomiting, weight gain. **Derm:** Rashes. **Misc:** Physical dependence, psychological dependence, tolerance.

Interactions: *Alcohol, antidepressants, other benzodiazepines, antihistamines, and opioid analgesics*-concurrent use results in ↑ CNS depression. *Hormonal contraceptives, disulfiram, fluoxetine, isoniazid, metoprolol, propoxyphene, propranolol, valproic acid, CYP3A4 inhibitors (erythromycin, ketoconazole, itraconazole, fluvoxamine, cimetidine, nefazodone)* ↓ metabolism of alprazolam, ↑ blood levels, and ↑ its actions (dose adjustments may be necessary). May ↓ efficacy of *levodopa*. *CYP3A4 inducers (rifampin, carbamazepine, or barbiturates)* ↑ metabolism and ↓ effects of alprazolam. Sedative effects may be ↓ by *theophylline*. *Cigarette smoking* ↓ blood levels and effects. ***Drug-Natural:*** *Kava-kava, valerian, or chamomile can* ↑ CNS depression. ***Drug-Food:*** Concurrent ingestion of *grapefruit juice* ↑ blood levels.
Dosage: **PO (Adults):** *Anxiety:* 0.25–0.5 mg 2–3 times daily (not >4 mg/day); *Panic attacks:* 0.5 mg 3 times daily; may ↑ by 1 mg or less every 3–4 days (not >10 mg/day). *Geriatric:* Start 0.25 mg 2–3 times daily. *Extended-release tablets (Xanax XR):* 0.5–1 mg once daily in the morning, may ↑ every 3–4 days (not more than 1 mg/day); up to 10 mg/day (usual range 3–6 mg/day). May need to dose XR twice daily for prophlyactic relief of anxiety/panic symptoms.
Availability (generic available)
Tablets: 0.25 mg, 0.5 mg, 1 mg, 2 mg. *Extended-release tablets:* 0.5 mg, 1 mg, 2 mg, 3 mg. *Orally disintegrating tablets (orange):* 0.25 mg, 0.5 mg, 1 mg, 2 mg. COST: Generic **$$**, Brand **$$$**

- **Geriatric Considerations:** Must reduce dose; assess for falls; ↑ risk for excessive CNS effects. Elderly have ↑ sensitivity to benzodiazepines.
- **Pediatric/Adolescent Considerations:** Safety and efficacy not established. ↓ dosage and frequent monitoring required.
- **Substance Abuse Considerations:** Addiction Severity Index; careful with personality disorders; high potential for abuse; high street resale value.
- **Clinical Assessments:** Monitor CBC, liver, renal function in long-term treatment. Monitor BP, pulse, respirations. Monitor for dizziness, lightheadedness.

DRUGS A-C

Clinical Tips/Alerts: Discontinue slowly, no more than 0.5 mg every 3 days to avoid withdrawal symptoms [mimics anxiety, panic attacks, pain in chest] (seizures have occurred); slower is better. Seizures may occur within first 3 days if stopped abruptly; requires slow reverse taper to discontinue. May have to taper along with longer-acting clonazepam. *Rule of thumb:* Every year of dependence = 1 month of tapering (3 years = 3 months).

Amitriptyline
(a-mee-**trip**-ti-leen) Elavil, Endep, *Apo-Amitriptyline, Levate, Novotriptyn*

Classification: *Therapeutic:* Antidepressants; *Pharmacological:* Tricyclic antidepressant; *Pregnancy Category C*

Indications: Depression. **Off-Label Use:** Anxiety, insomnia, treatment-resistant depression. Headaches, chronic pain syndromes (e.g., fibromyalgia, neuropathic pain/chronic pain).

Action: Potentiates effect of serotonin and norepinephrine in the CNS. Has significant anticholinergic properties.

Pharmacokinetics: *Absorption:* Well absorbed from GI tract. *Distribution:* Widely distributed. *Metabolism and Excretion:* Extensively metabolized by liver. Some metabolites have antidepressant activity. Undergoes enterohepatic recirculation and secretion into gastric juices. Probably crosses placenta and enters breast milk.

Protein Binding: 95% bound to plasma proteins.
$T_{1/2}$: 10–50 hr.

TIME/ACTION PROFILE (antidepressant effect)

Route	Onset	Peak	Duration
PO	2–3 wk (up to 30 days)	2–6 wk	Days-weeks
IM	2–3 wk	2–6 wk	Days-weeks

Contraindicated in: Angle-closure glaucoma; known history of QTc prolongation, recent myocardial infarction (MI), heart failure.

Use Cautiously in: Treatment of children or adolescents: monitor closely for suicidality; clients with pre-existing CV disease; benign prostatic hyperplasia (BPH) (↑ risk of urinary retention); history of seizures (threshold may be ↑) : **Pregnancy:** Use only if clearly needed and maternal benefits outweigh risk to fetus. *Lactation:* May cause sedation in infant.

Adverse Reactions/Side Effects (CAPITALS indicate life-threatening; <u>underlines</u> indicate most frequent)

CNS: <u>Lethargy</u>, <u>sedation</u>. **EENT:** <u>Blurred vision</u>, <u>dry eyes</u>, <u>dry mouth</u>. **CV:** ARRHYTHMIAS, <u>hypotension</u>, electrocardiogram (ECG) changes. **GI:** <u>Constipation</u>, hepatitis, paralytic ileus, ↑ appetite, weight gain. **GU:** Urinary retention, ↓ libido. **Derm:** Photosensitivity. **Endo:** Changes in blood glucose, gynecomastia. **Hemat:** Blood dyscrasias.

Interactions: Amitriptyline may be affected by drugs that compete for metabolism by cytochrome P450 2D6 enzyme, including other *antidepressants, phenothiazines, carbamazepine, class 1C antiarrhythmics* including *propafenone* and *flecainide;* when used concurrently with amitriptyline, dosage reduction of one or the other or both may be necessary. Other drugs that inhibit the activity of the enzyme, including *cimetidine, quinidine, amiodarone,* and *ritonavir,* may result in ↑ effects of amitriptyline. Concurrent use with *SSRI antidepressants* may result in ↑ toxicity and should be avoided (*fluoxetine* should be stopped 5 wk before starting amitriptyline). Concurrent use with *clonidine* may result in hypertensive crisis and should be avoided. Concurrent use with *levodopa* may result in delayed or ↓ absorption of levodopa or hypertension. Blood levels and effects may be ↓ by *rifamycins (rifampin, rifapentine,* and *rifabutin).* Concurrent use with *moxifloxacin* ↑ risk of adverse CV reactions. ↑ CNS depression with other *CNS depressants* including *alcohol, antihistamines, clonidine, opioids,* and *sedatives/hypnotics. Barbiturates* may alter blood levels and effects. *Adrenergic* and *anticholinergic* side effects may be ↑ with other agents having *anticholinergic* properties. *Phenothiazines* or *oral contraceptives* ↑ levels and may cause toxicity. *Nicotine* may ↑ metabolism and alter effects. ***Drug-Natural:*** St. John's wort may ↑ serum concentrations and efficacy. Concomitant use of *kava-kava, valerian, or chamomile* can ↑ CNS depression. ↑ Anticholinergic effects with *Jimson weed* and *scopolia.*

Dosage: PO (Adults): 75 mg/day in divided doses; may be ↑ up to 150 mg/day *or* 50–100 mg at bedtime; may ↑ by 25–50 mg up to 150 mg (hospitalized clients, may start with 100 mg/day, up to 300 mg/day). **PO (Geriatric Clients and Adolescents):** 10 mg 3 times daily and 20 mg at bedtime *or* 25 mg at bedtime initially, slowly ↑ to 100 mg/day as a single bedtime dose or divided doses.

Availability (generic available)

Tablets: 10 mg, 25 mg, 50 mg, 75 mg, 100 mg, 150 mg; **Syrup:** 10 mg/5 mL. COST: *Generic* **$**

DRUGS
A-C

- **Geriatric Considerations:** ↑ Risk of adverse reactions including falls due to sedative/anticholinergic effects.
- **Pediatric/Adolescent Considerations:** Safety not established in children <12 yr. Monitor closely (face to face), especially early in treatment for suicidality.
- **Clinical Assessments:** If history of CV disease or high doses: Monitor ECG before and throughout treatment. Monitor BP (reclining, standing, sitting) and pulse: watch for drop in BP or ↑ pulse.

Clinical Tips/Alerts: Drug overdose can result in death; monitor closely for suicidality and prescribe in smaller amounts. Do not use with alcohol. Adverse side effects (H₁): sedation, weight gain, hypotension; *cholinergic:* dry mouth, blurred vision, etc; often result in stopping of drug. May produce life-threatening arrhythmias; has resulted in sudden death. Potentially fatal reactions when used with *MAOIs* (avoid concurrent use–discontinue 2 wk before starting amitriptyline). Do not use with fluoxetine or clonidine (see *interactions*).

Amphetamine Mixtures

(am-**fet**-a-meen) Amphetamine Salt, Adderall, Adderall XR

Classification: *Therapeutic:* CNS stimulants
Schedule II; Pregnancy Category C

Indications: ADHD, children (ages ≥3 yr); ADHD, adults (Adderall XR): narcolepsy.

Action: Causes release of norepinephrine from nerve endings. Pharmacological effects are CNS and respiratory stimulation, vasoconstriction, mydriasis (pupillary dilation).

Pharmacokinetics: *Absorption:* Well absorbed after oral administration.

Distribution: Widely distributed in body tissues, with high concentrations in brain and cerebrospinal fluid (CSF). Crosses placenta and enters breast milk.

Metabolism and Excretion: Some metabolism by liver. Urinary excretion pH-dependent. Alkaline urine promotes reabsorption and prolongs action.

$T_{1/2}$: Children 6–12 yr: 9–11 hr; Adults: 10–13 hr (depends on urine pH).

Contraindicated in: Hyperexcitable states including hyperthyroidism; psychotic personalities; suicidal or homicidal tendencies; chemical dependence; glaucoma; structural cardiac abnormalities (may ↑ risk of sudden death); *Pregnancy:* Potentially embryotoxic.

TIME/ACTION PROFILE (CNS stimulation)

Route	Onset	Peak	Duration
PO	Tablet: 0.5–1 hr	Tablet: 3 hr Capsule: 7 hr	4–6 hr

Use Cautiously in: CV disease (sudden death has occurred in children with structural cardiac abnormalities or other serious heart problems); history of substance abuse (misuse may result in serious CV events/sudden death); hypertension; diabetes mellitus; Tourette's syndrome (may exacerbate tics).

Adverse Reactions/Side Effects (CAPITALS indicate life-threatening; underlines indicate most frequent)

CNS: Hyperactivity, insomnia, irritability, restlessness, tremor, dizziness, headache. **CV:** Palpitations, tachycardia, cardiomyopathy (↑ with prolonged use, high doses), hypertension, hypotension. **GI:** Anorexia, constipation, cramps, diarrhea, dry mouth, metallic taste, nausea, vomiting. **GU:** Erectile dysfunction, ↑ libido. **Derm:** Urticaria. **Endo:** Growth inhibition (with long-term use in children). **Misc:** Psychological dependence.

Interactions: Use with *MAOIs,* or *meperidine* can result in hypertensive crisis. ↑ Adrenergic effects with other *adrenergics or thyroid preparations. Drugs that alkalinize urine (sodium bicarbonate, acetazolamide)* ↓ excretion, ↑ effects. *Drugs that acidify urine (ammonium chloride,* large doses of *ascorbic acid)* ↑ excretion, ↓ effects, ↑ risk of hypertension and bradycardia with *beta blockers.* ↑ Risk of arrhythmias with *digoxin. Tricyclic antidepressants* may ↑ effect of amphetamine but may ↑ risk of arrhythmias, hypertension, or hyperpyrexia. *Drug-Natural:* Use with *St. John's wort* may ↑ serious side effects (avoid concurrent use). *Drug-Food:* Foods that alkalinize urine (fruit juices) can ↑ effect of amphetamine.

Dosage: Dose expressed in total amphetamine content (amphetamine + dextroamphetamine).

ADHD: PO (Children ≥6 yr): 5 mg/day 1–2 times daily; ↑ daily dose by 5 mg at weekly intervals. SR capsules can be given once daily, tablets every 8–12 hr. If starting therapy with extended-release capsules, start with 10 mg once daily and ↑ by 10 mg/day at weekly intervals (up to 60 mg/day).

PO (Adults): 20 mg/day initially (as extended-release product) up to maximum of 60 mg/day.

PO (Children 3–5 yr): 2.5 mg/day in the morning; ↑ daily dose by 2.5 mg at weekly intervals not to exceed 40 mg/day.

Availability *(generic available)*

Amount expressed in total amphetamine content (amphetamine + dextroamphetamine)

Tablets: 5 mg, 7.5 mg, 10 mg, 12.5 mg, 15 mg, 20 mg, 30 mg. *Extended-release capsules:* 5 mg, 10 mg, 15 mg, 20 mg, 25 mg, 30 mg. COST: Generic **$–$$** Brand (XR) **$$–$$$**

- **Geriatric Considerations:** More susceptible to adverse reactions.
- **Pediatric/Adolescent Considerations:** Monitor for weight loss, reduction in appetite. May have drug-free "holidays" (weekends, summers, school breaks) when using for inattentive-type ADHD. Do not use with known cardiac abnormalities.
- **Substance Abuse Considerations:** High potential for abuse; prolonged use may lead to dependence. Dispense sparingly; observe for obtaining for nontherapeutic use or distribution to others.
- **Clinical Assessments:** Monitor BP, pulse, and respiration before and during treatment, monitor height periodically. Monitor for rebound depression/fatigue when medication wears off.

Clinical Tips/Alerts: May cause sudden death with misuse or serious CV adverse events. Do not use with MAOIs or meperidine (see *Interactions*).

Aripiprazole

(a-ri-**pip**-ra-zole) Abilify

Classification: *Therapeutic:* Atypical antipsychotics, mood stabilizers

Pharmacological: Dihydrocarbostyril; Pregnancy Category C

Aripiprazole

21

Indications: Schizophrenia (age ≥13). Acute mania, mixed mania, bipolar disorder, maintenance of mood stabilization. Adjunct treatment of depression in adults. Adjunct treatment in bipolar and mixed mania (ages 10-17 yr), bipolar mania (ages 10-17 yr).

Action: Psychotropic activity may be due to agonist activity at dopamine D_2 and serotonin 5-HT_{1A} receptors and antagonist activity at the 5-HT_{2A} receptor. Also has alpha-1 adrenergic blocking activity.

Pharmacokinetics: *Absorption:* Well absorbed (87%) following oral administration; 100% following IM injection.

Distribution: Extensive extravascular distribution.

Metabolism and Excretion: Mostly metabolized by liver (CYP3A4 and CYP2D6 enzymes); one metabolite (dehydro-aripiprazole) has antipsychotic activity. 18% excreted unchanged in feces; <1% excreted unchanged in urine. Small percentage of clients poor metabolizers and may need smaller doses.

Protein Binding: *Aripiprazole and dehydro-aripiprazole:* >99%.

$T^{1}/_{2}$: *Aripiprazole:* 75 hr; *dehydro-aripiprazole:* 94 hr.

TIME/ACTION PROFILE (antipsychotic effect)

Route	Onset	Peak	Duration
PO	Unknown	2 wk	Unknown
IM	Unknown	1–3 hr	Unknown

Contraindicated in: Hypersensitivity. *Lactation:* Presumed to be excreted in breast milk; discontinue drug or bottle-feed.

Use Cautiously in: Known CV or cerebrovascular disease; conditions that cause hypotension (dehydration, treatment with antihypertensives or diuretics); concurrent ketoconazole or other potential CYP3A4 inhibitors (reduce aripiprazole dose by 50%); concurrent quinidine, fluoxetine, paroxetine, or other potential CYP2D6 inhibitors; concurrent carbamazepine or other potential CYP3A4 inducers; *Pregnancy:* Use only if benefit outweighs risk to fetus.

Adverse Reactions/Side Effects (CAPITALS indicate life-threatening; <u>underlines</u> indicate most frequent)

CNS: Akathisia, confusion, depression, <u>drowsiness,</u> <u>extrapyramidal reactions,</u> fatigue, hostility, insomnia, lightheadedness, manic reactions, impaired cognitive function, nervousness, restlessness, seizures, suicidal thoughts, tardive dyskinesia

(TD). **Resp:** Dyspnea. **CV:** Bradycardia, chest pain, edema, hypertension, orthostatic hypotension, tachycardia. **EENT:** Blurred vision, conjunctivitis, ear pain. **GI:** Constipation, anorexia. ↑ salivation, nausea, vomiting, weight loss. **GU:** Urinary incontinence. **Hemat:** Anemia. **Derm:** Dry skin, ecchymosis, skin ulcer, sweating. **MS:** Muscle cramps, neck pain. **Neuro:** Abnormal gait, tremor. **Misc:** NEUROLEPTIC MALIGNANT SYNDROME. ↓ heat regulation.

Interactions: Ketoconazole or other potential CYP3A4 *inhibitors* ↓ metabolism and ↑ effects (reduce aripiprazole dose by 50%). *Quinidine, fluoxetine, paroxetine, or other potential CYP2D6 inhibitors* ↓ metabolism and ↑ effects (reduce aripiprazole dose by at least 50%). ↑ Risk of serotonin syndrome with concurrent SSRI/SNRI antidepressants. Concurrent *carbamazepine or other potential CYP3A4 inducers* (double aripiprazole dose; then ↑ to 10–15 mg/day when interfering drug withdrawn.)

Dosage: *Schizophrenia:* **PO (Adults):** *Starting and target dose:* 10 or 15 mg/day as a single dose; doses up to 30 mg/day have been used; increments in dosing should not be made before 2 wk at a given dose.

PO (Adults and Children 13–17 yr): *Starting and target dose:* 2 mg/day as a single dose, then titrated up for 5 days to a target dose of 10 mg/day. Maximum dose 30 mg/day.

IM (Adults): 9.75 mg/day; may use a dose of 5.25 mg/day based on clinical situation. May give additional doses up to 30 mg if needed for agitation.

Bipolar mania: **PO (Adults):** 30 mg once daily; some clients may require 15 mg/day if 30 mg/day not tolerated. **IM (Adults):** 9.75 mg/day; may use dose of 5.25 mg based on clinical situation. May give additional doses up to 30 mg if needed for agitation. **PO (Children 10–17 yr):** Starting dose 2 mg/day; titrate up over 5 days to target dose of 10 mg/day. Maximum dose 30 mg/day. *Depression:* **PO, IM (Adults):** 2–5 mg/day; may titrate upward at 1-wk intervals to 5–10 mg/day, not to exceed 15 mg/day.

Availability

Tablets: 2 mg, 5 mg, 10 mg, 15 mg, 20 mg, 30 mg. **Tablets, orally disintegrating:** 10 mg, 15 mg. **Oral solution (orange cream):** 1 mg/mL. **Injection:** 9.75 mg/1.3 mL in ready-to-use vials. **COST:** Brand only $$$$

● **Geriatric Considerations:** ↑ Mortality in elderly with dementia-related psychosis.
● **Pediatric/Adolescent Considerations:** Now with safety profile in children ≥13 yr. Monitor for ↑ restlessness and changes in weight (BMI).

- **Clinical Assessments:** Monitor BMI (every month × 3, then every 90 d), monitor weight and measure waist circumference; fasting blood sugar, lipid profile; monitor BP. Better to prevent weight gain. (See *BMI/Metabolic Syndrome, Tools tab*.)

[**Clinical Tips/Alerts:** Be aware of long half-life and washout (see *Interactions*); least likely of antipsychotics to cause weight gain or diabetes.]

Atomoxetine

(a-to-**mox**-e-teen) Strattera

Classification: *Therapeutic:* Agents for ADHD; *Pharmacological:* SNRIs; *Pregnancy Category C*

Indications: ADHD in children ≥6 yr and adults.

Action: Selectively inhibits presynaptic reuptake transporter of norepinephrine.

Pharmacokinetics: *Absorption:* Well absorbed following oral administration. *Distribution:* Unknown. *Metabolism and Excretion:* Mostly metabolized by liver (CYP2D6 enzyme pathway). Small percentage of population poor metabolizers and has higher blood levels with ↑ effects).

Protein Binding: 98%.

T $\frac{1}{2}$: 5 hr.

TIME/ACTION PROFILE

Route	Onset	Peak	Duration
PO	Unknown	1–2 hr	12–24 hr

Contraindicated in: Concurrent with or within 2 wk therapy with MAOIs; angle-closure glaucoma.

Use Cautiously in: Hypertension, tachycardia, CV or cerebrovascular disease; pre-existing psychiatric illness; may ↑ risk of suicide attempt/ideation, especially during dose early treatment or dose adjustment; risk may be greater in children or adolescents; concurrent albuterol or vasopressors (↑ risk of adverse CV reactions); *Pregnancy:* Use only if benefits outweigh risks to fetus; *Lactation:* Safety not established.

Adverse Reactions/Side Effects (CAPITALS indicate life-threatening; underlines indicate most frequent)

CNS: Dizziness, fatigue, mood swings. **Adults:** Insomnia. **CV:** Hypertension, orthostat-ic hypotension, tachycardia. **GI:** Dyspepsia, severe liver injury (rare), nausea, vomiting. **Adults:** Dry mouth, constipation. **Derm:** Rash, urticaria. **GU: Adults:** Dysmenorrhea, ejaculatory problems, ↓ libido, erectile dysfunction, urinary hesitation, urinary retention. **Metab:** ↑ Appetite, weight/growth loss. **Misc:** ALLERGIC REACTIONS INCLUDING ANGIONEUROTIC EDEMA.

Interactions: Concurrent use with *MAOIs* may result in serious, potentially fatal reac-tions (do not use within 2 wk of each other). ↑ Risk of CV effects with *albuterol* or *vasopressors* (use cautiously). *Drugs that inhibit CYP2D6 enzyme pathway (quinidine, fluoxetine, paroxetine)* will ↑ blood levels and effects, dose ↓ recommended.

Dosage: PO (Children and adolescents <70 kg): 0.5 mg/kg/day initially; may be ↑ every 3 days to a daily target dose of 1.2 mg/kg given as a single dose in the morn-ing or evenly divided doses in the morning and late afternoon/early evening (not to exceed 1.4 mg/kg/day or 100 mg/day, whichever is less). *If taking concurrent CYP2D6 inhibitor (quinidine, fluoxetine, paroxetine):* 0.5 mg/kg/day initially; may ↑ if needed to 1.2 mg/kg/day after 4 wk.

PO (Adults, adolescents, and children >70 kg): 40 mg/day initially; may be ↑ every 3 days to a daily target dose of 80 mg/day given as a single dose in the morn-ing or evenly divided doses in the morning and late afternoon/early evening; may be further ↑ after 2–4 wk to 100 mg/day. *If taking concurrent CYP2D6 inhibitor (quinidine, fluoxetine, paroxetine):* 40 mg/day initially; may ↑ if needed to 80 mg/day after 4 wk.

Hepatic Impairment: PO (Adults and Children): *Moderate hepatic impairment (Child; Pugh Class B):* ↓ Initial and target dose by 50%; *severe hepatic impairment (Child; Pugh Class C):* ↓ initial and target dose to 25% of normal.

Availability

Capsules: 10 mg, 18 mg, 25 mg, 40 mg, 60 mg, 80 mg, 100 mg. COST: Brand only **$$$**

Geriatric Considerations: Caution with hypertension, CV, cerebrovascular disease.

● **Pediatric/Adolescent Considerations:** ↑ Risk of suicidal ideation; monitor closely. Potential for severe liver injury has been reported in children and adults. May be prudent to check liver functions periodically.

● **Clinical Assessments:** Take a thorough medical history and perform physical exam (ECG, echocardiogram); exertional chest pain or syncope requires immediate cardiac evaluation. Assess for hepatic injury (jaundice, dark urine, right upper quadrant [RUQ] tenderness, etc.)

[**Clinical Tips/Alerts:** Due to potential risk of hepatotoxicity, periodic monitoring of liver function tests (LFTs) in children and adults warranted. **]**

Benztropine

(**benz**-troe-peen) Cogentin, *Apo-Benztropine*

Classification: *Therapeutic:* Antiparkinson/anti-EPS agents; *Pharmacological:* Anticholinergics; *Pregnancy Category C*

Indications: Adjunctive treatment of all forms of Parkinson's disease, including drug-induced extrapyramidal effects (akinesia, akathisia, rabbit syndrome) and acute dystonic reactions. Does not treat TD.

Action: Blocks cholinergic activity in CNS, which is partially responsible for symptoms of Parkinson's disease. Restores natural balance of neurotransmitters in CNS.

Pharmacokinetics: *Absorption:* Well absorbed following PO and IM administration. *Distribution:* Unknown. *Metabolism and Excretion:* Unknown.

T $\frac{1}{2}$: Unknown.

TIME/ACTION PROFILE (antidyskinetic activity)

Route	Onset	Peak	Duration
PO	1–2 hr	Several days	24 hr
IM, IV	Within minutes	Unknown	24 hr

Contraindicated in: Hypersensitivity; children <3 yr; angle-closure glaucoma; TD.
Use Cautiously in: Prostatic hyperplasia; seizure disorders; cardiac arrhythmias; *Pregnancy/Lactation:* Safety not established.
Adverse Reactions/Side Effects: (CAPITALS indicate life-threatening; underlines indicate most frequent)
CNS: Confusion, depression, dizziness, hallucinations, headache, sedation, weakness. **EENT:** Blurred vision, dry eyes, mydriasis. **CV:** Arrhythmias, hypotension, palpitations, tachycardia. **GI:** Constipation, dry mouth, ileus, nausea. **GU:** Hesitancy, urinary retention. **Misc:** ↑ Sweating.

Interactions: Additive anticholinergic effects with *drugs sharing anticholinergic properties,* such as antihistamines, phenothiazines, quinidine, disopyramide, and *tri-cyclic antidepressants.* Counteracts cholinergic effects of bethanechol. Antacids and antidiarrheals may ↓ absorption. *Drug-Natural:* ↑ Anticholinergic effect with *angel's trumpet, Jimson weed,* and *scopolia.*

Dosage: *Parkinsonism:* **PO (Adults):** 1–2 mg/day in one to two divided doses (range 0.5–6 mg/day). *Acute dystonic reactions:* **IM, IV (Adults):** 1–2 mg, then 1–2 mg PO twice daily. *Drug-induced extrapyramidal reactions:* **PO, IM, IV (Adults):** 1–4 mg given once or twice daily (1–2 mg 2–3 times daily may also be used PO).

Availability (generic available).
Tablets: 0.5 mg, 1 mg, 2 mg. **Injection:** 1 mg/mL. COST: Generic **$**

- **Geriatric Considerations:** Elderly have ↑ risk of adverse reactions and are sensitive to anticholinergics (constipation, urinary retention [BPH])
- **Pediatric/Adolescent Considerations:** Safety not established, although anecdotal reports show efficacy in decreasing EPS symptoms related to antipsychotic medication therapy.
- **Clinical Assessments:** Monitor input and output (I&O). Monitor for urinary retention (dysuria, infrequent voiding) and constipation. ↑ Fluids and fiber intake (fruits, vegetables, supplements).

Clinical Tips/Alerts: Confusion or hallucinations may be sign of toxicity, as well as nausea, vomiting, hyperthermia. Be especially careful during hot weather and use in alcoholics; may result in heat stroke and hyperthermia. Taper slowly unless needed for serious adverse event, such as toxicity; abrupt withdrawal can cause anxiety, insomnia, tachycardia, return of EPS. (See *EPS, Basics tab.*)

BuPROPion HCl

(byoo-**proe**-pee-on) Wellbutrin, Wellbutrin SR, Wellbutrin XL, Zyban; buPROPion HBr: Aplenzin

Classification: *Therapeutic:* Antidepressants, smoking cessation
Pharmacological: Aminoketones; *Pregnancy Category B*

Indications: Treatment of major depression (immediate release [IR], sustained release [SR], extended release [XL]). Depression in seasonal affective disorder (XL only). Smoking cessation (Zyban only). **Off-Label Use:** Treatment of ADHD in adults

(SR only). Sexual dysfunction and ↓ libido in men and women. ↓ Addictive behaviors (food cravings, drug binging).

Action: ↓ Neuronal reuptake of dopamine and norepinephrine in CNS. Buproprion is a norepinephrine dopamine reuptake inhibitor (NDRI).

Pharmacokinetics: *Absorption:* Although well absorbed, rapidly and extensively metabolized by liver. *Distribution:* Unknown.

Metabolism and Excretion: Extensively metabolized by liver. Some conversion to active metabolites.

T $^1/_2$: 14 hr (active metabolites may have longer half-lives).

TIME/ACTION PROFILE (antidepressant effect)

Route	Onset	Peak	Duration
PO	1–3 wk	Unknown	Unknown

Contraindicated in: Hypersensitivity; history of bulimia, and anorexla nervosa; concurrent MAOI or ritonavir therapy; *Lactation:* Secreted in breast milk; potential for serious adverse reactions in nursing infants. Discontinue nursing or discontinue drug. **Use Cautiously in:** Renal/hepatic impairment (↓ dose recommended); recent history of MI; history of suicide attempt; unstable CV status; children and adolescents; *Pregnancy:* Use only if benefit to client outweighs potential risk to fetus. *Use Extreme Caution in:* History of seizures, head trauma, or concurrent medications that ↓ seizure threshold (theophylline, antipsychotics, antidepressants, systemic corticosteroids); severe hepatic cirrhosis (↓ dose required); children and adolescents.

Adverse Reactions/Side Effects: (CAPITALS indicate life-threatening; <u>underlines</u> indicate most frequent)

CNS: SEIZURES, <u>agitation,</u> <u>headache,</u> insomnia, mania, psychoses. **GI:** <u>Dry mouth, nausea,</u> <u>vomiting,</u> change in appetite, weight gain, weight loss. **Derm:** Photosensitivity. **Endo:** Hyperglycemia, hypoglycemia, syndrome of inappropriate antidiuretic hormone (SIADH) secretion. **Neuro:** <u>Tremor.</u>

Interactions: ↑ Risk of adverse reactions when used with *amantadine, levodopa,* or *MAOIs* (concurrent use of MAOIs contraindicated). ↑ Risk of seizures with *phenothiazines, antidepressants, theophylline, corticosteroids, OTC stimulants/anorectics,* or cessation of *alcohol* or *benzodiazepines* (avoid or minimize alcohol use). Blood levels ↑ by *ritonavir* (avoid concurrent use). *Carbamazepine* may ↓ blood levels and effectiveness. *Concurrent use with nicotine replacement* may cause hypertension.

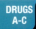

↑ Risk of bleeding with *warfarin*. Bupropion and one of its metabolites inhibit CYP2D6 enzyme system and may ↑ levels and risk of toxicity from *antidepressants* (SSRIs and tricyclic), some *beta blockers, antiarrhythmics, and antipsychotics.*

Dosage: *Depression: PO (Adults): IR:* 100 mg twice daily initially; after 3 days may ↑ up to 100 mg 3 times daily; after at least 4 wk of therapy, may ↑ up to 450 mg/day in divided doses (not to exceed 150 mg/dose; wait at least 6 hr between doses at 300 mg/day dose or at least 4 hr between doses at 450 mg/day dose). *SR:* 150 mg once daily in the morning; after 3 days, may ↑ to 150 mg twice daily with at least 8 hr between doses; after at least 4 wk of therapy, may ↑ to a maximum daily dose of 400 mg given as 200 mg twice daily. *XL:* 150 mg once daily in the morning, may be ↑ after 4 days to 300 mg once daily; some clients may require up to 450 mg/day as a single daily dose. *Bupropion HBr (Aplenzin) (Adults):* Start 174 mg every morning; after 4 days ↑ to 348 mg; maximum 522 mg/day.

Seasonal Affective Disorder: PO (Adults): 150 mg/day in the morning; if dose well tolerated, ↑ to 300 mg/day in 1 wk. Doses should be tapered to 150 mg/day for 2 wk before discontinuing.

Smoking cessation: PO (Adults): *Zyban:* 150 mg once daily for 3 days, then 150 mg twice daily for 7–12 wk (doses should be at least 8 hr apart).

Availability (generic available)

Tablets: 75 mg, 100 mg. COST: *Generic* $. **SR tablets:** 100 mg, 150 mg, 200 mg; COST: *Generic* $$. **XL tablets:** 150 mg, 300 mg. COST: *Generic* $$$. **Bupropion HBr XL tablets:** 174 mg, 348 mg, 522 mg. Cost $$$.

● **Geriatric Considerations:** Be aware of possible drug accumulation (↓ kidney clearance); ↑ sensitivity to adverse effects. Preferable to start with a lower dose.

● **Pediatric/Adolescent Considerations:** ↑ Risk of suicidal behavior; monitor closely (face to face) early on in treatment and during dosage adjustments. Use with caution.

● **Clinical Assessments:** Monitor for suicidality, seizure activity, changes in mood (up or down). In liver/renal disease, monitor hepatic/renal functions.

● **Clinical Tips/Alerts:** Seizure risk ↑ fourfold at doses >450 mg, especially with IR and SR preparations; caution with bipolar disorder (use bupropion with concomitant mood stabilizer), avoid alcohol. Equally space out doses to reduce chance of seizures; do not exceed 150 mg/dose (see *Dosage*). Do not use if severe insomnia exists. Do not administer bupropion with Zyban. **FDA approval** (4/23/2009): Once-daily formulation of bupropion HBr (Aplenzin) as extended-release tablets for major depressive disorder.

BusPIRone

(byoo-**spye**-rone) BuSpar

Classification: *Therapeutic:* Antianxiety agents; *Pregnancy Category B*

Indications: Management of anxiety; generalized anxiety disorder or short-term relief of anxiety; anxiety associated with depression.

Action: Binds to serotonin and dopamine receptors in brain. ↑ Norepinephrine metabolism in brain.

Pharmacokinetics: *Absorption:* Rapidly absorbed. *Distribution:* Unknown. *Metabolism and Excretion:* Extensively metabolized by liver (CYP3A4 enzyme system); 20%–40% excreted in feces.

Protein Binding: 95% bound to plasma proteins.

T $1/2$: 2–3 hr.

TIME/ACTION PROFILE (relief of anxiety)

Route	Onset	Peak	Duration
PO	7–10 days	3–4 wk	Unknown

Contraindicated in: Hypersensitivity; severe hepatic or renal impairment; concurrent use of MAOIs; ingestion of large amounts of grapefruit juice.

Use Cautiously in: Clients receiving other antianxiety agents (other agents should be withdrawn slowly to prevent withdrawal or rebound phenomenon); clients receiving other psychotropics; *Lactation/Pregnancy:* Safety not established.

Adverse Reactions/Side Effects: (CAPITALS indicate life-threatening; underlines indicate most frequent)

CNS: Dizziness, drowsiness, excitement, fatigue, headache, insomnia, nervousness, weakness, personality changes. **EENT:** Blurred vision, nasal congestion, sore throat, tinnitus, altered taste or smell, conjunctivitis. **Resp:** Chest congestion, hyperventilation, shortness of breath. **CV:** Chest pain, palpitations, tachycardia, hypertension, hypotension, syncope. **GI:** Nausea, abdominal pain, constipation, diarrhea, dry mouth, vomiting. **GU:** Changes in libido, dysuria, urinary frequency, urinary hesitancy. **Derm:** Rashes, alopecia, blisters, dry skin, easy bruising, edema, flushing, pruritus. **Endo:** Irregular menses. **MS:** Myalgia. **Neuro:** Incoordination, numbness, paresthesia, tremor. **Misc:** Clamminess, sweating, fever.

BusPIRone/Carbamazepine

Interactions: Use with *MAOIs* may result in hypertension and not recommended. *Erythromycin, nefazodone, ketoconazole, itraconazole, ritonavir,* and other inhibitors *of CYP3A4* ↑ blood levels and effects of buspirone; dose reduction recommended (↓ to 2.5 mg twice daily with erythromycin, ↓ to 2.5 mg once daily with nefazodone). *Rifampin, dexamethasone, phenytoin, phenobarbital, carbamazepine,* and other inducers *of CYP3A4* ↓ blood levels and effects of buspirone; dose adjustment may be necessary. Avoid concurrent use with *alcohol.*
Drug-Natural: Concomitant use of *kava, valerian, or chamomile* can ↑ CNS depression. **Drug-Food:** *Grapefruit juice* ↑ serum levels and effect; ingestion of large amounts of grapefruit juice not recommended.

Dosage: **PO (Adults):** 7.5 mg twice daily; ↑ by 5 mg/day every 2–4 days as needed (not to exceed 60 mg/day). Usual dose 20–30 mg/day (in two divided doses).

Availability (generic available)
Tablets: 5 mg, 7.5 mg, 15 mg, 30 mg. COST: *Generic $*

● **Geriatric Considerations:** Does not cause usual sedation or cognitive impairments of other antianxiety drugs (see *Clinical Tips/Alerts*).
● **Pediatric/Adolescent Considerations:** Safety not established. Has shown ↑ in aggressive behaviors in children with Pervasive Developmental Disorders.
● **Clinical Assessments:** Monitor hepatic/renal function with impairment. Monitor for reduction of anxiety. Does not seem to cause physical/psychological dependence.

Clinical Tips/Alerts: Buspirone not effective as a PRN (as needed) medication and requires consistent dosing. Be aware that 15- and 30-mg tabs (called Dividose Tabs) are divided into three scored segments that allow for dosage adjustments (e.g., 30 mg would equal entire tab, 20 mg would equal 2/3 tab, and 10 mg would equal 1/3 tab). Elderly living alone may not be able to comprehend dividing tabs for dosing or physically able to break tabs.

Carbamazepine
(Kar-ba-**maz**-e-peen) Tegretol, Carbatrol, Epitol, Equetro, Tegretol-XR, Teril
Apo-Carbamazepine, Novo-Carbamaz, Tegretol CR
Classification: *Therapeutic:* Anticonvulsants (second generation), mood stabilizers;
Pregnancy Category D

Indications: Treatment of tonic-clonic, mixed, and complex-partial seizures; pain in trigeminal neuralgia or diabetic neuropathy. **Equetro only:** Acute mania and mixed episodes, bipolar I disorder. **Off-Label Use:** Other forms of neurogenic pain, aggressive behaviors, mood dysregulation.

Action: ↓ Synaptic transmission in CNS by affecting sodium channels in neurons. Inhibits release of glutamate.

Pharmacokinetics: *Absorption:* Absorption slow but complete. Suspension produces earlier higher peak and lower trough levels.

Distribution: Widely distributed. Crosses blood-brain barrier. Crosses placenta rapidly and enters breast milk in high concentrations.

Metabolism and Excretion: Extensively metabolized in liver by cytochrome P4503A4 to active epoxide metabolite; epoxide metabolite has anticonvulsant and antineuralgic activity.

Protein Binding: *Carbamazepine:* 75%–90%; *epoxide:* 50%.

T $1/2$: *Carbamazapine:* single dose: 25–65 hr; Chronic dosing: *children:* 8–14 hr; *adults:* 12–17 hr; *epoxide:* 34 ± 9 hr.

TIME/ACTION PROFILE (anticonvulsant activity)

Route	Onset	Peak	Duration
PO	Up to 1 mo†	4–5 hr‡	6–12 hr
PO–ER	Up to 1 mo†	2–3–12 hr‡	12 hr

†Onset of antineuralgic activity 8–72 hr. ‡Listed for tablets; peak level occurs 1.5 hr after chronic dose of suspension.

Contraindicated in: Hypersensitivity; bone-marrow suppression; concomitant use or use within 14 days of MAOIs; *Pregnancy:* Use only during pregnancy if potential benefits outweigh risks to fetus; additional vitamin K during last weeks of pregnancy has been recommended; *Lactation:* Discontinue drug or bottle-feed.

Use Cautiously in: Cardiac or hepatic disease; renal failure (dosing adjustment required for CCr <10 mL/min); ↑ intraocular pressure; older men with prostatic hyperplasia.

Adverse Reactions/Side Effects: (CAPITALS indicate life-threatening; underlines indicate most frequent)

CNS: ataxia, drowsiness, fatigue, psychosis, sedation, vertigo. **EENT:** Blurred vision, nystagmus, corneal opacities. **Resp:** Pneumonitis. **CV:** CHF, edema, hypertension, hypotension, syncope. **GI:** Hepatitis, pancreatitis, weight gain. **GU:** Hesitancy, urinary

Derm: Photosensitivity, rashes, STEVENS-JOHNSON SYNDROME (SJS), TOXIC EPIDERMAL NECROLYSIS (TEN), urticaria. **Endo:** SIADH, hyponatremia. **Hemat:** AGRANULOCYTOSIS, APLASTIC ANEMIA, THROMBOCYTOPENIA, eosinophilia, leukopenia. **Misc:** Chills, fever, lymphadenopathy, elevated liver enzymes, multiorgan hypersensitivity reactions, hepatic failure (rare).

Interactions: May ↑ metabolism of and therefore ↓ levels/effectiveness of corticosteroids, doxycycline, felbamate, quinidine, warfarin, estrogen-containing contraceptives, barbiturates, cyclosporine, benzodiazepines, theophylline, lamotrigine, phenytoin, topiramate, valproic acid, bupropion, and haloperidol. Danazol ↑ blood levels (avoid concurrent use if possible). Concurrent use (within 2 wk) of MAOIs may result in hyperpyrexia, hypertension, seizures, and death. Verapamil, diltiazem, propoxyphene, itraconazole, ketoconazole, erythromycin, clarithromycin, SSRIs, antidepressants, and cimetidine may inhibit hepatic metabolism or carbamazepine and ↑ levels; may cause toxicity. Enzyme inducers such as rifampin, phenobarbital, phenytoin, primidone, and methosuximide may ↑ serum concentration of carbamazepine. May ↑ risk of hepatotoxicity from isoniazid. Felbamate ↓ carbamazepine levels but ↑ levels of active metabolite. May ↓ effectiveness and ↑ risk of toxicity from acetaminophen. May ↑ risk of CNS toxicity from lithium. May ↑ duration of action of nondepolarizing neuromuscular blocking agents.

Drug-Food: Grapefruit juice ↑ serum levels and oral bioavailability by 40% and therefore may ↑ effects.

Dosage: PO (Adults): Bipolar (Equetro): 400 mg/day in divided doses, twice daily. ↑ by 200 mg/day every 3–4 days until optimal clinical response, up to 1600 mg/day. Anticonvulsant: 200 mg twice daily (tablets) or 100 mg 4 times daily (suspension); ↑ by 200 mg/day every 7 days until therapeutic levels achieved (range 600–1200 mg/day in divided doses every 6–8 hr; not to exceed 1 g/day in 12–15-yr-olds. Extended-release products given twice daily (XR, CR). Antineuralgic: 100 mg twice daily or 50 mg 4 times daily (suspension); ↑ by up to 200 mg/day until pain is relieved, then maintenance dose of 200–1200 mg/day in divided doses (usual range 400–800 mg/day).

PO (Children 6–12 yr): 100 mg twice daily (tablets) or 50 mg 4 times daily (suspension); ↑ by 100 mg weekly until therapeutic levels obtained (usual range 400–800 mg/day; not to exceed 1 g/day). Extended-release products (XR, CR) given twice daily.

PO (Children <6 yr): 10–20 mg/kg/day in two to three divided doses; may be ↑ at weekly intervals until optimal response and therapeutic levels achieved. Usual maintenance dose 250–350 mg/day (not to exceed 35 mg/kg/day).

Availability (generic available).
Tablets: 200 mg. COST: *Generic* **$. Chewable tablets:** 100 mg; Canada: 200 mg. COST: *Generic* **$. XR capsules:** 100 mg, 200 mg, 300 mg. COST: **$$. XR tablets:** 100 mg, 200 mg, 400 mg. COST: **$–$$. Oral suspension (citrus/vanilla flavor):** 100 mg/5 mL; COST: *Generic* **$.**

● **Geriatric Considerations:** Use with caution in men with BPH (↑ urinary retention); because of sedation, monitor for dizziness/falls.

● **Pediatric/Adolescent Considerations:** Approved for use in epilepsy, therefore safety profile exists. Used off-label for aggression.

● **Clinical Assessments:** Before treatment, detailed physical and medical history; *baseline tests:* CBC, platelets with differential; perform ECG; liver, kidney, thyroid function tests. Then *monitor* CBC, platelets, and differntial weekly × 2 months, then two to three times a year during treatment. Monitor serum electrolytes: possible *hyponatremia. Monitor* for signs of bruising, bleeding, fever, sore throat, infections (*aplastic anemia, thrombocytopenia*). *Monitor* for signs of serious dermatological reaction-*SJS:* Fever, skin rash, blisters on skin or mucous membranes, hives, swollen tongue. SJS and TEN happen in 1-6 per 10,000 new users (mostly Caucasian); Asian risk 10 times higher; Chinese ancestry with HLA-B*1502 associated with greater risk (populations genetically at risk should be screened for HLA-B*1502). Those of Asian ancestry, including South Asian Indians, should be tested for HLA-B*1502 before being prescribed carbamazapine (FDA Alert, 12/12/2007: www.fda.gov/cder/drug/InfoSheets/HCP/carbamazepineHCP.htm). Those testing positive should not be prescribed carbamazapine. *Monitor* for mood changes and suicidality.

Clinical Tips/Alerts: If a rash develops, discontinue carbamazapine until medically evaluated for SJS (see *Clinical Assessments*). If client is of Asian ancestry, see *Clinical Assessments*. Carbamazapine requires baseline and ongoing monitoring (see *Clinical Assessments*) because of possible serious and life-*threatening side effects. Discontinue if bone-marrow* depression occurs. Do not use concurrently with MAOI. **Equetro** consists of three types of beads: immediate-, extended-, and enteric-release to provide twice-daily dosing. Do not crush or chew.

Chlordiazepoxide

(Klor-dye-az-e-**pox**-ide) Libritabs, Librium, Librax (in combination w/clidinium), Limbitrol DS (in combination w/amytriptyline), Apo-Chlordiazepoxide, Mitran, Novopoxide, Poxi

Classification: *Therapeutic:* Antianxiety agents, sedatives/hypnotics; *Pharmacological:* Benzodiazepines; *Schedule IV; Pregnancy Category D*

Indications: Adjunct management of anxiety. Treatment of alcohol withdrawal. Adjunct management of anxiety associated with acute myocardial infarction.

Action: Acts at many levels of CNS to produce anxiolytic effect. Depresses CNS, probably by potentiating GABA, an inhibitory neurotransmitter.

Pharmacokinetics: *Absorption:* Well absorbed from GI tract. IM absorption may be slow and unpredictable.

Distribution: Widely distributed. Crosses blood-brain barrier. Crosses placenta; enters breast milk. Recommend to discontinue drug or bottle-feed.

Metabolism and Excretion: Highly metabolized by liver. Some products of metabolism are active as CNS depressants.

$T^{1}/_{2}$: 5–30 hr.

TIME/ACTION PROFILE (sedation)

Route	Onset	Peak	Duration
PO	1–2 hr	0.5–4 hr	Up to 24 hr
IM	15–30 min	Unknown	Unknown
IV	1–5 min	Unknown	0.25–1 hr

Contraindicated in: Hypersensitivity; some products contain tartrazine and should be avoided in clients with known intolerance; cross-sensitivity with other benzodiazepines may occur; comatose clients or those with pre-existing CNS depression; uncontrolled severe pain; pulmonary disease; angle-closure glaucoma; porphyria; children ≤6 yr.

Pregnancy/Lactation: May cause CNS depression, flaccidity, feeding difficulties, and weight loss in infants; discontinue nursing or drug.

Use Cautiously in: Hepatic dysfunction; severe renal impairment; history of suicide attempt or substance abuse; elderly (sedation).

Adverse Reactions/Side Effects: (CAPITALS indicate life-threatening; underlines indicate most frequent)

CNS: <u>Dizziness,</u> <u>drowsiness,</u> hangover, headache, mental depression, paradoxical excitation, sedation. **EENT:** Blurred vision. **GI:** Constipation, diarrhea, nausea, vomiting, weight gain. **Derm:** Rashes. **Local:** <u>Pain at IM site.</u> **Misc:** Physical dependence, psychological dependence, tolerance.

Interactions: *Alcohol, antidepressants, antihistamines,* and *opioid analgesics:* concurrent use results in additive CNS depression. *Cimetidine, oral contraceptives, disulfiram, fluoxetine, isoniazid, ketoconazole, metoprolol, propoxyphene, propranolol, or valproic acid* may enhance effects. May ↓ efficacy of *levodopa. Rifampin* or **barbiturates** may ↓ effectiveness of chlordiazepoxide. Sedative effects may be ↓ by *theophylline.* **Drug-Natural:** Concomitant use of *kava, valerian, chamomile, or hops* can ↑ CNS depression.

Dosage: PO (Adults): *Alcohol withdrawal:* 50–100 mg, repeated until agitation is controlled (up to 400 mg/day). *Anxiety:* 5–25 mg 3–4 times daily around the clock. **PO (Geriatric or Debilitated Clients):** *Anxiety:* 5 mg 2–4 times daily initially, ↑ as needed. **PO (Children >6yr):** *Anxiety:* 5 mg 2–4 times daily (up to 10 mg 2–3 times daily). **IM, IV (Adults):** *Alcohol withdrawal:* 50–100 mg initially; may be repeated in 2–4 hr. *Anxiety:* 50–100 mg initially, then 25–50 mg 3–4 times daily as required (25–50 mg initially in geriatric clients). *Preoperative sedation:* 50–100 mg 1 hr preoperative. **IM, IV (Geriatric or Debilitated Clients):** *Anxiety/sedation:* 25–50 mg/dose. **IM, IV (Children >12 yr):** *Anxiety/sedation:* 25–50 mg/dose.

Availability (generic available)

Capsules: 5 mg, 10 mg, 25 mg. **Tablets:** 5 mg, 10 mg, 25 mg. **Injection:** 100 mg ampule. COST: **$.** *In combination with:* amitriptyline (Limbitrol DS), clidinium (Librax).

- **Geriatric Considerations:** Long-acting benzodiazepines cause prolonged sedation in elderly. Appears on Beers list and is associated with ↑ risk of falls (↓ dose required or consider short-acting benzodiazepine); debilitated clients (initial dose reduction required).
- **Pediatric/Adolescent Considerations:** Not for use in children ≤6 yr.
- **Substance Abuse Considerations:** Possible risk for dependency with history of alcohol or drug abuse.
- **Clinical Assessments:** Monitor anxiety level/reduction; CBCs and LFTs on prolonged therapy.

DRUGS A–C

[**Clinical Tips/Alerts:** Injectable form used for alcohol withdrawal; assess for seizures.

ChlorproMAZINE

(Klor-**proe**-ma-zeen) Thorazine, Thor-Prom, Chlorpromanyl, Largactil, Novo-Chlorpromazine

Classification: *Therapeutic:* Antiemetics, antipsychotics; *Pharmacological:* Phenothiazines (low potency); *Pregnancy Category UK*

Indications: Schizophrenia and psychoses. Hyperexcitable, combative, explosive behavior in children. Hyperactive child with conduct disorder. Acute mania. Nausea and vomiting. Intractable hiccups. Preoperative apprehension. Acute intermittent porphyria. **Off-Label Use:** Vascular headache. Bipolar disorder.

Action: Alters effects of dopamine (D_2) in CNS. Has significant anticholinergic/alpha-adrenergic blocking activity.

Pharmacokinetics: *Absorption:* Variable absorption from tablets/suppositories; better with oral liquid formulations. Well absorbed following IM administration. *Distribution:* Widely distributed; high CNS concentrations. Crosses placenta; enters breast milk. *Metabolism and Excretion:* Highly metabolized by liver and GI mucosa. Some metabolites are active.

Protein Binding: ≥90%.

T $1/_2$: 30 hr.

TIME/ACTION PROFILE (antipsychotic activity, antiemetic activity, sedation)

Route	Onset	Peak	Duration
PO	30–60 min	Unknown	4–6 hr
PO-ER	30–60 min	Unknown	10–12 hr
Rectal	1–2 hr	Unknown	3–4 hr
IM	Unknown	Unknown	4–8 hr
IV	Rapid	Unknown	Unknown

Contraindicated in: Hypersensitivity; hypersensitivity to sulfites (injectable) or benzyl alcohol (SR capsules); cross-sensitivity with other phenothiazines may occur; angle-closure glaucoma; bone-marrow depression; severe liver/CV disease; concurrent pimozide use.

Chlordiazepoxide/Chlorpromazine

36

Use Cautiously in: Diabetes; respiratory disease; prostatic hyperplasia; CNS tumors; epilepsy; intestinal obstruction; dehydrated or sick children. *Pregnancy/Lactation:* Safety not established. Discontinue drug or bottle-feed.

Adverse Reactions/Side Effects: (CAPITALS indicate life-threatening; underlines indicate most frequent)

CNS: NEUROLEPTIC MALIGNANT SYNDROME, sedation, extrapyramidal reactions, TD. **EENT:** Blurred vision, dry eyes, lens opacities. **CV:** Hypotension (↑ with IM, IV), tachycardia. **GI:** Constipation, dry mouth, anorexia, hepatitis, ileus, priapism. **GU:** Urinary retention. **Derm:** Photosensitivity, pigment changes, rashes. **Endo:** Galactorrhea, amenorrhea. **Hemat:** AGRANULOCYTOSIS, leukopenia. **Metab:** Hyperthermia. **Misc:** Allergic reactions.

Interactions: Concurrent use with *pimozide* ↑ risk of potentially serious CV reactions. May alter serum *phenytoin* levels. ↓ Pressor effect of *norepinephrine* and eliminates bradycardia. Antagonizes peripheral vasoconstriction from *epinephrine* and may reverse some of its actions. May ↓ elimination and ↑ effects of *valproic acid*. May ↓ pharmacological effects of *amphetamine* and *related compounds*. May ↓ effectiveness of *bromocriptine*. May ↑ blood levels and effects of *tricyclic antidepressants*. *Antacids* or *adsorbent antidiarrheals* may ↓ adsorption; administer 1 hr before or 2 hr after chlorpromazine. *Activated charcoal* ↓ absorption. ↑ Risk of anticholinergic effects with *antihistamines, tricyclic antidepressants, quinidine,* or *disopyramide*. Premedication with chlorpromazine ↑ risk of neuromuscular excitation and hypotension when followed by *barbiturate* anesthesia. *Barbiturates* may ↑ metabolism and ↓ effectiveness. Chlorpromazine may ↓ *barbiturate* blood levels. Additive hypotension with *antihypertensives*. Additive CNS depression with *alcohol, antidepressants, antihistamines, MAOIs, opioid analgesics, sedatives/hypnotics,* or *general anesthetics*. Concurrent use with *lithium* may produce disorientation, unconsciousness, or extrapyramidal symptoms. Concurrent use with *meperidine* may produce excessive sedation and hypotension. May ↑ risk of seizures with subarachnoid *metrizamide*. Concurrent use with *propranolol* ↑ blood levels of both drugs. *Drug-Natural:* Concomitant use of *kava, valerian, chamomile, or hops* can ↑ CNS depression. ↑ Anticholinergic effects with *angel's trumpet, Jimson weed, and scopolia*.

Dosage: **PO (Adults):** *Psychoses:* 10–25 mg 2–4 times daily; may ↑ every 3–4 days (usual dose is 200 mg/day; up to 1 g/day) *or* 30–300 mg 1–3 times daily as extended-release capsules.

PO (Children ≥1 yr): *Severe behavior problems:* 0.55 mg/kg every 4–6 hr PRN, maximum dose: 40 mg/day. **PO Children:** *Psychoses/nausea and vomiting:* 0.55 mg/kg (15 mg/m²) every 4–6 hr as needed.

IM (Adults): *Severe psychoses:* 25–50 mg initially, may be repeated in 1 hr; ↑ to maximum of 400 mg every 3–12 hr if needed (up to 1 g/day).

IM (Children ≥1 yr): *Severe behavior problems:* 0.55 mg/kg every 6–8 hr PRN. Maximum dose: 40 mg/day (≤5 yr); 75 mg/day (ages 5–12 yr).

IM (Children >6 mo): *Psychoses/nausea and vomiting:* 0.55 mg/kg (15 mg/m²) every 6–8 hr (not to exceed 40 mg/day in children 6 mo–5 yr, or 75 mg/day in children 5–12 yr).

Availability (generic available)
Tablets: 10 mg, 25 mg, 50 mg, 100 mg, 200 mg. **SR capsules:** 30 mg, 75 mg, 150 mg, 200 mg, 300 mg. **Syrup (orange custard flavor):** 10 mg/5 mL; Canada: 25 mg/5 mL; 100 mg/5 mL. **Oral concentrate (custard flavor):** 30 mg/mL; Canada: 40 mg/mL, 100 mg/mL. **Suppositories:** 25 mg, 100 mg. **Injection:** 25 mg/mL. COST: $

● **Geriatric Considerations:** ↑ Initial dose in elderly/debilitated clients. Use cautiously with CV and chronic respiratory diseases. ↑ Risk of mortality in elderly with dementia-related psychosis.

● **Pediatric/Adolescent Considerations:** Children with acute illnesses, infections, gastroenteritis, or dehydration (↑ risk of extrapyramidal reactions).

● **Clinical Assessments:** Take a baseline weight and FBS, cholesterol panel, and BMI; monitor weight, BMI, FBS, and cholesterol. (See *BMI/Metabolic Syndrome, Tools tab*.) Consider alternative antipsychotic with obese/diabetic client. Monitor BP, pulse, respirations, evaluate for hypotension and tachycardia. Monitor for elevated prolactin levels resulting in sexual side effects, galactorrhea, polydipsia. Monitor for EPS, TD, and neuroleptic malignant syndrome (NMS). (See *Psychotropic Adverse Effects, Basics tab.*)

Clinical Tips/Alerts: Very sedating conventional antipsychotic; should be used only for short-term treatment/management and is considered a second-line treatment after atypicals. Conventional antipsychotics reduce positive signs of schizophrenia (hallucinations) but are not as effective with negative signs (apathy).

Citalopram

(si-**tal**-oh-pram) Celexa

Classification: *Therapeutic*: Antidepressants; *Pharmacological*: SSRIs; *Pregnancy Category C*

Indications: Depression. **Off-Label Use:** PMDD. OCD. Panic disorder. GAD. Post-traumatic stress disorder (PTSD). Social anxiety disorder (social phobia).

Action: Selectively inhibits reuptake of serotonin in CNS.

Pharmacokinetics: *Absorption:* 80% absorbed after oral administration. *Distribution:* Enters breast milk. *Metabolism and Excretion:* Mostly metabolized by liver (10% by CYP 3A4 and 2C19 enzymes); excreted unchanged in urine.

T $\frac{1}{2}$: 35 hr.

TIME/ACTION PROFILE (antidepressant effect)

Route	Onset	Peak	Duration
PO	1–4 wk	Unknown	Unknown

Contraindicated in: Hypersensitivity; concurrent MAOI or pimozide therapy.

Use Cautiously in: History of mania; history of suicide attempt/ideation ($\uparrow$ risk during early therapy and during dose adjustment); history of seizure disorder; illnesses or conditions that are likely to result in altered metabolism or hemodynamic responses; severe renal or hepatic impairment; in children and adolescents. *Pregnancy:* Use during third trimester may result in neonatal serotonin syndrome requiring prolonged hospitalization and respiratory and nutritional support; *Lactation:* Citalopram present in breast milk and may result in lethargy with $\uparrow$ feeding in infants; weigh risk/benefits.

Adverse Reactions/Side Effects: (CAPITALS indicate life-threatening; <u>underlines</u> indicate most frequent)

CNS: <u>Apathy,</u> <u>confusion,</u> <u>drowsiness,</u> <u>insomnia,</u> <u>weakness,</u> agitation, amnesia, anxiety, $\downarrow$ libido, dizziness, fatigue, impaired concentration, $\uparrow$ depression, migraine headache, suicide attempt. **EENT:** Abnormal accommodation. **Resp:** Cough. **CV:** Postural hypotension, tachycardia. **GI:** <u>Abdominal pain,</u> <u>anorexia,</u> <u>diarrhea,</u> <u>dry mouth,</u> <u>dyspepsia,</u> <u>flatulence,</u> $\uparrow$ <u>saliva,</u> <u>nausea,</u> altered taste, $\uparrow$ appetite, vomiting. **GU:** Amenorrhea, dysmenorrhea, ejaculatory delay, erectile dysfunction, polyuria. **Derm:** ↑ Sweating, photosensitivity, pruritus, rash. **Metab:** ↓ Weight, ↑ weight. **MS:** Arthralgia, myalgia. **Neuro:** Tremor, paresthesia. **Misc:** Fever, yawning.

Interactions: May cause serious, potentially fatal reactions when used with *MAOIs;* allow at least 14 days between citalopram and *MAOIs.* Concurrent use with *pimozide* may result in prolongation of QTc interval and is contraindicated. Use cautiously with other *centrally acting drugs* (including *alcohol, antihistamines, opioid analgesics,* and *sedatives/hypnotics);* concurrent use with *alcohol* not recommended). *Cimetidine* ↑ blood levels of citalopram. Serotonergic effects may be ↑ by *lithium* (concurrent use should be carefully monitored). *Ketoconazole, itraconazole, erythromycin,* and *omeprazole* may ↑ blood levels. *Carbamazepine* may ↓ blood levels. May ↑ blood levels of *metoprolol.* Concurrent use with *tricyclic antidepressants* should be undertaken with caution because of altered pharmacokinetics. Concurrent use with *5-HT₁ agonists* for migraine headaches may ↑ risk of adverse reactions (weakness, hyperreflexia, incoordination). Use cautiously with *tricyclic antidepressants* due to unpredictable effects on serotonin and norepinephrine reuptake. Risk of bleeding may be ↑ with *aspirin, NSAIDs, warfarin, thrombolytics,* and other *agents affecting coagulation and platelet function. Drug-Natural:* ↑ risk of serotonergic side effects including serotonin syndrome with St. John's wort and *SAMe.*

Dosage: PO (Adults): 20 mg once daily initially, may be ↑ by 20 mg/day at weekly intervals up to 60 mg/day (usual dose 40 mg/day).

PO (Geriatric Clients): 20 mg once daily initially, may be ↑ to 40 mg/day only in non-responding clients. **Hepatic Impairment: PO (Adults):** 20 mg once daily initially, may be ↑ to 40 mg/day only in nonresponding clients.

Availability (generic available)

Tablets: 10 mg, 20 mg, 40 mg. COST: *Generic $.* **Oral solution (peppermint flavor):** 10 mg/5 mL. COST: *Generic $.*

● **Geriatric Considerations:** Recommend reduced dose. Lower dose with hepatic/renal impairment.

● **Pediatric/Adolescent Considerations:** May ↑ risk of suicide attempt/ideation, especially during early treatment or dose adjustment in children/adolescents (off label for pediatric use); monitor closely for suicidality (face to face) initially, then during dosage adjustments.

● **Clinical Assessments:** Assess for improvement in mood as well as suicidality. Be vigilant if mood improves greatly and client starts giving possessions away or reconnecting with previous relationships.

Clinical Tips/Alerts: Be aware of potential for suicide with mood improvement (energy to carry out act). *Ask client if he/she has thoughts of suicide. Assess for risk:* Speaks of suicide, has a plan, gives possessions away, current loss or multiple losses, does not see a future or purpose in life, isolation, stressful events, substance abuse, lethal method available. May cause serious, potentially fatal reactions when used with *MAOIs*; allow at least 14 days between citalopram and *MAOIs*. (See *Serotonin Syndrome, Basics tab.*) Do not use concurrently with *pimozide.*

ClomiPRAMINE

(kloe-**mip**-ra-meen) Anafranil

Classification: *Therapeutic:* Antiobsessive agents; *Pharmacological:* Tricyclic antidepressants; *Pregnancy Category C*

Indications: OCD. **Off-Label Use:** Depression, neuropathic pain/chronic pain.

Action: Potentiates effect of serotonin (antiobsessional effect) and norepinephrine in CNS. Has moderate anticholinergic effect.

Pharmacokinetics: *Absorption:* Well absorbed from GI tract.

Distribution: Widely distributed, enters breast milk. *Metabolism and Excretion:* Extensively metabolized by liver. Some conversion to a pharmacologically active metabolite (desmethylclomipramine). Undergoes enterohepatic recirculation and secretion into gastric juices.

Protein Binding: ≥90%.

T ½: 21–31 hr.

TIME/ACTION PROFILE

Route	Onset	Peak	Duration
PO	1–6 wk	Unknown	Unknown

Contraindicated in: Hypersensitivity; Angle-closure glaucoma; recent myocardial infarction; history of QTc prolongation; cardiac arrythmias; heart failure; concurrent MAOI or clonidine use (avoid if possible); **Pregnancy:** Potential for fetal harm or neonatal withdrawal syndrome. **Lactation:** Discontinue drug or bottle-feed.

Use Cautiously in: History of seizures (threshold may be lowered); clients with pre-existing CV disease; older men with prostatic hyperplasia (may be more susceptible to urinary retention); hyperthyroidism (↑ risk of arrhythmias); may ↑ risk of suicide attempt/ideation, especially during dose early treatment or dose adjustment.

Adverse Reactions/Side Effects: (CAPITALS indicate life-threatening; underlines indicate most frequent)

CNS: SEIZURES; lethargy, sedation, weakness, aggressive behavior. **EENT:** Blurred vision, dry eyes, dry mouth, vestibular disorder. **CV:** ARRHYTHMIAS, ECG changes, orthostatic hypotension. **GI:** Constipation, nausea, vomiting, weight gain, eructation. **GU:** Male sexual dysfunction, urinary retention. **Derm:** Dry skin, photosensitivity. **Endo:** Gynecomastia. **Hemat:** Anemia. **MS:** Muscle weakness. **Neuro:** Extrapyramidal reactions. **Misc:** Hyperthermia.

Interactions: May cause hypotension and tachycardia when used with MAOIs (concurrent use not recommended). Wait 2 wk before initiating clomipramine after MAOIs are stopped. Wait 2 wk before initiating MAOIs after clomipramine is stopped. May prevent therapeutic response to antihypertensives. Use with clonidine may result in hypertensive crisis (avoid concurrent use). ↑ CNS depression with other CNS depressants including alcohol, antihistamines, opioids, and sedatives/hypnotics. Adrenergic and anticholinergic side effects may be ↑ with other agents having adrenergic/anticholinergic properties. Effects and toxicity may be ↑ by concurrent use with SSRI antidepressants (wait several weeks after stopping SSRIs to start clomipramine; up to 5 weeks for fluoxetine), phenothiazines, cimetidine, or oral contraceptives. Nicotine may ↑ metabolism and ↓ effectiveness. Transient delirium may occur with disulfiram. **Drug-Natural:** ↑ Risk of serotonergic side effects including serotonin syndrome with St. John's wort and SAMe. Kava, valerian, and chamomile can ↑ CNS depression. **Drug-Food:** Grapefruit juice ↑ serum levels and effect.

Dosage: PO (Adults): Antiobsessive: 25 mg/day, ↑ over 2 wk to 100 mg/day in divided doses. May be further ↑ over several weeks up to 250-300 mg/day in divided doses. Once stabilizing dose reached, entire daily dose may be given at bedtime. Antidepressant: 25 mg 3 times daily, may be ↑ as needed (unlabeled). **PO (Geriatric Clients):** 20-30 mg/day initially, may be ↑ as needed. **PO (Children >10-17 yr):**

25 mg/day initially, ↑ over 2 wk to 3 mg/kg/day or 100 mg/day (whichever is smaller) in divided doses. May be further ↑ to 3 mg/kg/day or 200 mg/day (whichever is smaller) in divided doses. Once stabilizing dose reached, entire daily dose may be given at bedtime.

Availability (generic available)

Capsules: 10 mg, 25 mg, 50 mg, 75 mg. COST: **$**

- **Geriatric Considerations:** ↑ risk of arrhythmias. BPH: more susceptible to urinary retention.
- **Pediatric/Adolescent Considerations:** Safety not established in children <10 yr. ↑ risk of suicide; monitor closely (face to face) initially and then during dosage adjustments.
- **Clinical Assessments:** Assess for reduction in either obsessive thoughts or compulsions. Associated with weight gain: Perform baseline BMI, weight, FBS, and cholesterol panel. (See *BMI/Metabolic Syndrome, Tools tab*.)

Clinical Tips/Alerts: This was one of the first OCD psychotropics; often SSRI antidepressants (e.g., fluoxetine) are now used because of side-effect profile of clomipramine. Do not use with history of QTc interval prolongation or cardiac disease.

Clonazepam

(kloe-**na**-ze-pam) Klonopin, *Rivotril, Syn-Clonazepam*

Classification: *Therapeutic:* Anticonvulsants; *Pharmacological:* Benzodiazepines; Schedule IV; Pregnancy Category D

Indications: Prophylaxis of: Petit mal, petit mal variant, akinetic, myoclonic seizures. Panic disorder with or without agoraphobia. **Off-Label Use:** Restless leg syndrome. Neuralgias. Sedation. Adjunct management of acute mania, acute psychosis, or insomnia.

Action: Anticonvulsant effects may be due to presynaptic inhibition. Produces sedative effects in CNS, probably by stimulating inhibitory GABA receptors in cerebral cortex.

Pharmacokinetics: *Absorption:* Well absorbed from GI tract. *Distribution:* Probably crosses blood-brain barrier and placenta. *Metabolism and Excretion:* Mostly metabolized by liver.

T $^1/_2$: 18–50 hr.

Clonazepam

TIME/ACTION PROFILE (anticonvulsant activity)

Route	Onset	Peak	Duration
PO	20–60 min	1–2 hr	6–12 hr

Contraindicated in: Hypersensitivity to clonazepam or other benzodiazepines; severe liver disease.

Use Cautiously in: Angle-closure glaucoma; obstructive sleep apnea; chronic respiratory disease; history of porphyria; do not discontinue abruptly. **Pregnancy:** Safety not established; chronic use during pregnancy may result in withdrawal in neonate; **Lactation:** May enter breast milk; discontinue drug or feed by bottle.

Adverse Reactions/Side Effects (CAPITALS indicate life-threatening; underlines indicate most frequent)

CNS: Behavioral changes, drowsiness, fatigue, slurred speech, ataxia, sedation, abnormal eye movements, diplopia, nystagmus. **Resp:** ↓ Secretions. **CV:** Palpitations. **GI:** Constipation, diarrhea, hepatitis, weight gain. **GU:** Dysuria, nocturia, urinary retention. **Hemat:** Anemia, eosinophilia, leukopenia, thrombocytopenia. **Neuro:** Ataxia, hypotonia. **Misc:** Fever, physical dependence, psychological dependence, tolerance.

Interactions: *Alcohol,* antihistamines, other benzodiazepines, and opioid analgesics: Concurrent use results in ↑ CNS depression. *Cimetidine,* hormonal contraceptives, disulfiram, fluoxetine, isoniazid, ketoconazole, metoprolol, propoxyphene, propranolol, and valproic acid may ↑ metabolism of clonazepam. ↑ its actions. May ↓ efficacy of levodopa. *Rifampin or barbiturates* may ↑ metabolism and ↓ effectiveness of clonazepam. Sedative effects may be ↓ by *theophylline.* May ↑ serum *phenytoin* levels. *Phenytoin* may ↑ serum clonazepam levels. **Drug-Natural:** Concomitant use of *kava, valerian, or chamomile* can ↑ CNS depression.

Dosage: PO (Adults): 0.5 mg 3 times daily; may ↑ by 0.5–1 mg every 3rd day. Total daily maintenance dose not to exceed 20 mg. *Panic disorder:* 0.125 mg twice daily; ↑ after 3 days toward target dose of 1 mg/day (some clients may require up to 4 mg/day).

PO (Children <10 yr or 30 kg): Initial daily dose 0.01–0.03 mg/kg/day (not to exceed 0.05 mg/kg/day) given in 2–3 equally divided doses; ↑ by no more than 0.25–0.5 mg every 3rd day until therapeutic blood levels reached (not to exceed 0.2 mg/kg/day).

Availability (generic available)
Tablets: 0.5 mg, 1 mg, 2 mg. COST: *Generic* **$. Orally disintegrating tablets:** 0.125 mg, 0.25 mg, 0.5 mg, 1 mg, 2 mg. COST: *Generic* **$$.**

- **Geriatric Considerations:** May experience excessive sedation at usual doses; ↓ dosage recommended.
- **Pediatric/Adolescent Considerations:** Indicated for absence seizures in children; no psychiatric child indications, use caution when dosing and discontinuing.
- **Substance Abuse Considerations:** Less abuse potential than other benzodiazepines. Good tolerability, less euphoria, abuse, dependence, and street value.
- **Clinical Assessments:** Monitor anxiety level/reduction; drowsiness, sedation (dose-dependent).

Clinical Tips/Alerts: Because of long half-life, considered a good choice for long-term treatment of anxiety. Although indication may allow for dosing up to 20 mg/day, in psychiatry dose is typically less than 8 mg/day. Monitor compliance to avoid withdrawal.

Clonidine

(**klon**-i-deen) Catapres, Catapres-TTS, Duraclon, *Dixarit*
Classification: *Therapeutic*: antihypertensives; *Pharmacological*: adrenergics (centrally acting); *Pregnancy Category C*
Indications: **PO, Transdermal:** Management of mild to moderate hypertension.
Off-Label Use: Attention deficit disorder, Tourette's syndrome, management of opioid and alcohol withdrawal, anxiety disorders.
Action: Stimulates alpha-adrenergic receptors in CNS, which results in ↑ sympathetic outflow, inhibiting cardioacceleration and vasoconstriction centers. Prevents pain signal transmission to CNS by stimulating alpha-adrenergic receptors in spinal cord.
Pharmacokinetics: *Absorption:* Well absorbed from GI tract and skin. Enters systemic circulation following epidural use. Some absorption follows sublingual administration. *Distribution:* Widely distributed; enters CNS. Crosses placenta readily; enters breast milk in high concentrations. *Metabolism and Excretion:* Mostly metabolized by liver; 40%–50% eliminated unchanged in urine.
Half-life: *Plasma:* 12–22 hr; *CNS:* 1–3 hr.

TIME/ACTION PROFILE (PO, TD = antihypertensive effect; epidural = analgesia)

Route	Onset	Peak	Duration
PO	30–60 min	2–4 hr	8–12 hr
Transdermal	2–3 days	Unknown	7 days*
Epidural	Unknown	Unknown	Unknown

*8 hr following removal of patch

Contraindicated in: Hypersensitivity; *Epidural:* Injection site infection, anticoagulant therapy, or bleeding problems.

Use Cautiously in: Serious cardiac or cerebrovascular disease; renal insufficiency; *Pregnancy or lactation:* Safety not established.

Adverse Reactions/Side Effects (CAPITALS indicate life-threatening; underlines indicate most frequent)

CNS: Drowsiness, depression, dizziness, nervousness, nightmares. **CV:** Bradycardia, hypotension (↑ with epidural), palpitations. **GI:** Dry mouth, constipation, nausea, vomiting. **GU:** Erectile dysfunction. **Derm:** Rash, sweating, **F and E:** Sodium retention. **Metab:** Weight gain. **Misc:** Withdrawal phenomenon.

Interactions: Additive sedation with *CNS depressants,* including *alcohol, antihistamines, opioid analgesics,* and *sedatives/hypnotics.* Additive hypotension with other *antihypertensives and nitrates.* Additive bradycardia with *myocardial depressants,* including *beta blockers, amphetamines, beta blockers, prazosin,* or *tricyclic antidepressants* may ↓ antihypertensive effect. Withdrawal phenomenon may be ↑ by discontinuation of *beta blockers.* Epidural clonidine prolongs effects of epidurally administered *local anesthetics.* May ↓ effectiveness of *levodopa.* ↑ Risk of adverse CV reactions with verapamil.

Dosage: **PO (Children):** (off label). *Tourettes. ADHD.* Start 0.05 mg at bedtime; ↑ by 0.025 or 0.05 mg in divided daily doses (2–4 times/day) every 3–4 days, until symptoms abate. *Maximum dose:* 100 mcg (0.1 mg) twice daily. ↑ by 100–200 mcg **PO (Adults):** *Hypertension (initial dose):* 100 mcg (0.1 mg) in 2–4 divided doses. *Usual maintenance dose* 200–600 mcg (0.2–0.6 (0.1–0.2 mg)/day every 2–4 days. *Usual maintenance dose* 200–600 mcg (0.2–0.6 mg)/day in two to three divided doses (up to 2.4 mg/day). *Urgent treatment:* 200 mcg (0.2 mg) loading dose, then 100 mcg (0.1 mg) every hour until BP controlled or 800 mcg (0.8 mg) total has been administered; follow with maintenance dosing. *Opioid withdrawal:* 300 mcg (0.3 mg)—1.2 mg/day; may be ↑ by 50%/day for 3 days, then discontinued or ↓ by 100–200 mcg (0.1–0.2 mg)/day. **PO (Geriatric Clients):** 100 mcg (0.1 mg) at bedtime initially, ↑ as needed. **PO (Children):** 50–400 mcg (0.05–0.4 mg) twice daily. **Transdermal (Adults):** *Hypertension:* Transdermal system delivering 100–300 mcg (0.1–0.3 mg)/24 hr applied every 7 days. Initiate with 100 mcg (0.1 mg)/24-hr system; dosage increments may be made every 1–2 wk when system is changed.

Availability (generic available)

Tablets: Canada: 25 mcg (0.025 mg), 100 mcg (0.1 mg), 200 mcg (0.2 mg), 300 mcg (0.3 mg). COST: *Generic* **$. Transdermal systems:** Catapres-TTS 1 releases 0.1 mg/24 hr; Catapres-TTS 2 releases 0.2 mg/24 hr; Catapres-TTS 3 releases 0.3 mg/24 hr. COST: Catapres-TTS **$$–$$$.**

● **Geriatric Considerations:** Appears on Beers list due to ↑ risk of orthostatic hypotension and adverse CNS effects in geriatric clients (↓ dose recommended).

● **Pediatric/Adolescent Considerations:** Due to drowsiness and sedation, titrate in increments of 0.025 mg-0.05 mg every 4–7 days.

● **Clinical Assessments:** Monitor BP with dose changes.

[**Clinical Tips/Alerts:** DO NOT STOP ABRUPTLY; must be tapered to discontinue due to potential for rebound hypertension.]

Clozapine

(**kloe**-za-peen) Clozaril, FazaClo

Classification: *Therapeutic:* Atypical antipsychotic; *Pregnancy Category B*

Indications: Schizoprenia unresponsive to or intolerant of standard therapy with other antipsychotics (treatment refractory). To reduce recurrent suicidal behavior in schizophrenic clients.

Action: Binds to dopamine receptors in CNS. Also has anticholinergic and alpha-adrenergic blocking activity. Produces fewer extrapyramidal reactions and less TD than standard antipsychotics but carries high risk of hematological abnormalities.

Pharmacokinetics: *Absorption:* Well absorbed after oral administration. *Distribution:* Rapid and extensive distribution; crosses blood-brain barrier and placenta.

Metabolism and Excretion: Mostly metabolized on first pass through liver.
Protein Binding: 95%.
T½ 8–12 hr.

TIME/ACTION PROFILE (antipsychotic effect)

Route	Onset	Peak	Duration
PO	Unknown	Weeks	4–12 hr

Contraindicated in: Hypersensitivity; bone-marrow depression; severe CNS depression/coma; uncontrolled epilepsy; granulocytopenia; **Lactation:** Discontinue drug or bottle-feed.
Use Cautiously in: Prostatic enlargement; angle-closure glaucoma; malnourished clients or clients with CV, hepatic, or renal disease (use lower initial dose, titrate more slowly); diabetes; seizure disorder. **Pregnancy:** Use only if clearly needed.

Adverse Reactions/Side Effects: (CAPITALS indicate life-threatening; underlines indicate most frequent)

CNS: NEUROLEPTIC MALIGNANT SYNDROME, SEIZURES, dizziness, sedation. **EENT:** Visual disturbances. **CV:** MYOCARDITIS, hypotension, tachycardia, ECG changes, hypertension. **GI:** Constipation, abdominal discomfort, dry mouth, ↑ salivation, nausea, vomiting, weight gain. **Derm:** Rash, sweating. **Endo:** Hyperglycemia. **Hemat:** AGRANU-LOCYTOSIS, LEUKOPENIA. **Neuro:** Extrapyramidal reactions. **Misc:** Fever.

Interactions: ↑ Anticholinergic effects with other agents having anticholinergic properties, including antihistamines, quinidine, disopyramide, and antidepressants. Concurrent use with SSRI antidepressants ↑ blood levels and risk of toxicity (especially fluvoxamine). ↑ CNS depression with alcohol, antidepressants, antihistamines, opioid analgesics, or sedative/hypnotics. ↓ Hypotension with nitrates, acute ingestion of alcohol, or antihypertensives. ↑ Risk of bone-marrow suppression with antihypertensives or radiation therapy. Use with lithium ↑ risk of adverse CNS reactions, including seizures.
Drug-Natural: Caffeine-containing herbs (cola nut, tea, coffee) may ↑ serum levels and side effects. St. John's wort may ↑ blood levels and efficacy.

Dosage: PO (Adults): 25 mg 1–2 times daily initially; ↑ by 25–50 mg/day over 2 wk up to target dose of 300–450 mg/day. May ↑ by up to 100 mg/day once or twice further (not to exceed 900 mg/day). Treatment should be continued for at least 2 yr in clients with suicidal behavior.

Availability (generic available)

Tablets: 25 mg, 100 mg. **Orally disintegrating tablets (mint):** 25 mg, 100 mg. COST: Generic **$$–$$$**

- **Geriatric Considerations:** ↑ Risk of death of elderly clients with dementia-related psychosis.
- **Pediatric/Adolescent Considerations:** Safety not established in children <16 yr.
- **Clinical Assessments:** Must follow Clozaril protocol: Monitor BP/pulse (sitting/standing); CBC (white blood cell/differential <3000/mm^3; withhold clozapine). Monitor for signs of myocarditis, akathisia, EPS, and NMS. (*See Psychotropic Adverse Effects, Tools tab.*) Monitor FBS, cholesterol, Hbg A$_1$C, weight, and BMI before and throughout therapy. (*See BMI/Metabolic Syndrome, Tools tab.*)

Clinical Tips/Alerts: Clozapine is an effective yet serious drug for treatment of treatment-resistant schizophrenia. Protocols must be followed because of serious/life-threatening side effects. Medication is supplied only in 1–wk amounts. [***See Clozaril Protocol, Labs/Protocols tab.***] Clozapine is known for ↑ in weight and possibility of diabetes and metabolic syndrome (↑ abdominal fat, hyperglycemia, ↑ lipids).

Psychotropic Drugs D–G

Desipramine

(dess-**ip**-ra-meen) Norpramin, Pertofrane

Classification: *Therapeutic:* Antidepressants; *Pharmacological:* Tricyclic antidepressants; *Pregnancy Category C*

Indications: Depression. **Off-Label Use:** Chronic pain syndromes. Anxiety. Insomnia.

Action: Potentiates effect of serotonin and norepinephrine in the CNS. Has significant anticholinergic properties.

Pharmacokinetics: *Absorption:* Well absorbed from GI tract.

Distribution: Widely distributed. *Metabolism and Excretion:* Extensively metabolized by liver. One metabolite is pharmacologically active (2-hydroxydesipramine). Undergoes enterohepatic recirculation and secretion into gastric juices. Small amounts enter breast milk.

Protein Binding: 90%–92%.

T 1/2: 12–27 hr.

TIME/ACTION PROFILE (antidepressant effect)

Route	Onset	Peak	Duration
PO	2–3 wk	2–6 wk	Days–weeks

Contraindicated in: Angle-closure glaucoma; recent MI, heart failure, known history of QTc prolongation.

Use Cautiously in: Clients with pre-existing CV disease; prostatic hyperplasia (↓ susceptibility to urinary retention); history of seizures (threshold may be ↓); may ↑ risk of suicide attempt/ideation esp. during early treatment or dose adjustment; risk may be greater in children or adolescents. *Pregnancy/Lactation:* Use during pregnancy only if potential maternal benefit outweighs risks to fetus; use during lactation may result in neonatal sedation.

Adverse Reactions/Side Effects: (CAPITALS indicate life-threatening; underlines indicate most frequent.)

CNS: Drowsiness, fatigue. **EENT:** Blurred vision, dry eyes, dry mouth. **CV:** ARRHYTH-MIAS, hypotension, ECG changes. **GI:** Constipation, drug-induced hepatitis, paralytic ileus, ↑ appetite, weight gain. **GU:** Urinary retention. **Derm:** Photosensitivity, ↑ libido. **Endo:** Changes in blood glucose, gynecomastia. **Hemat:** Blood dyscrasias.

Interactions: Desipramine metabolized in liver by cytochrome P450 2D6 enzyme and its action may be affected by drugs that compete for metabolism by or alter activity of this enzyme, including other *antidepressants, phenothiazines, carbamazepine, class 1C* antiarrhythmics *(propafenone, flecainide, encainide);* when used concurrently, dose reduction of one or the other or both may be necessary. Concurrent use of other drugs that inhibit activity of the enzyme, including *cimetidine, quinidine, amiodarone,* and *ritonavir,* may result in ↑ effects. May cause hypotension, tachycardia, and potentially fatal reactions when used with *MAOIs* (avoid concurrent use—discontinue 2 wk prior). Concurrent use with *SSRI antidepressants* may result in ↑ toxicity and should be avoided (fluoxetine should be stopped 5 wk before). Concurrent use with *clonidine* may result in hypertensive crisis and should be avoided. *Phenytoin* may ↓ levels and effectiveness; ↑ doses of desipramine may be required to treat depression. Concurrent use with *levodopa* may result in delayed/↓ absorption of levodopa or hypertension. Blood levels and effects may be ↓ by *rifamycins, carbamazepine,* and *barbiturates.* Concurrent use with *moxifloxacin* ↑ risk of adverse CV reactions. ↑ CNS depression with other *CNS depressants,* including *alcohol, antihistamines, clonidine, opioid analgesics,* and *sedatives/hypnotics.* *Barbiturates* may alter blood levels and effects. *Adrenergic* and *anticholinergic* side effects may be ↑ with other *agents having these properties. Hormonal contraceptives* ↑ levels and may cause toxicity. *Cigarette smoking* may ↑ metabolism and alter effects.

Drug-Natural: Concomitant use of *kava, valerian,* or *chamomile* can ↑ CNS depression. ↑ anticholinergic effects with *Jimson weed* and *scopolia.*

Dosage: PO (Adults): 100–200 mg/day as a single dose or in divided doses (up to 300 mg/day). **PO (Geriatric Clients):** 25–50 mg/day in divided doses (up to 150 mg/day). **PO (Children >12 yr):** 25–50 mg/day in divided doses, ↑ as needed up to 100 mg/day. **PO (Children 6–12 yr):** 10–30 mg/day (1–5 mg/kg/day) in divided doses.

Availability (generic available)

Tablets: 10 mg, 25 mg , 50 mg, 75 mg, 100 mg, 150 mg. COST: **$**

● **Geriatric Considerations:** ↑ sensitivity to drug effects: hypotension, drowsiness; risk of falls; caution with CV disease; contraindicated with MI, QTc prolongation, heart failure, BPH.

- **Pediatric/Adolescent Considerations:** Safety not established in children <12 yr. Monitor for sedation, dizziness, and ataxia. Risk for suicide greater in children/adolescents; monitor closely for suicidal ideation.
- **Clinical Assessments:** Monitor BP and pulse before/after Rx. Look for drop in BP or ↑ in pulse. History CV disease. ECG before and after Rx. Monitor weight and BMI (weight gain); monitor FBS, cholesterol if weight gain. (*See BMI/Metabolic Syndrome, Tools tab.*)

Clinical Tips/Alerts: Not a first-line option for depression; good for chronic pain.

Desvenlafaxine

(des-ven-la-**fax**-een) Pristiq

Classification: *Therapeutic:* Antidepressants; *Pregnancy Category C*

Indications: Major depressive disorder in adults.

Action: Inhibits serotonin and norepinephrine reuptake in CNS.

Pharmacokinetics: *Absorption:* 80% absorbed after oral administration. *Distribution :* Extensive distribution into body tissues. *Metabolism and Excretion:* Extensively metabolized on first pass through liver. One metabolite, O-desmethylvenlafaxine (ODV), has antidepressant activity; 45% of the active metabolite excreted unchanged in urine at 72 hours.

$T\frac{1}{2}$: 11 hr.

TIME/ACTION PROFILE (antidepressant action)

Route	Onset	Peak	Duration
PO	4–5 days	4–5 days	Unknown

Contraindicated in: Hypersensitivity; concurrent MAOI therapy.

Use Cautiously in: CV disease, including hypertension; hepatic impairment; impaired renal function; history of seizures or neurological impairment; history of mania; history of ↑ intraocular pressure or angle-closure glaucoma; observe closely for suicidality and behavior changes; history of drug abuse. **Pregnancy:** Use only if clearly required during pregnancy, weighing benefit to mother versus potential harm to fetus (potential for discontinuation syndrome or toxicity in neonate when taken during third trimester). *Lactation:* Potential for serious adverse reactions in infant; discontinue drug or discontinue breastfeeding.

Adverse Reactions/Side Effects: (CAPITALS indicate life-threatening; underlines indicate most frequent.)

CNS: SEIZURES, abnormal dreams, anxiety, dizziness, headache, insomnia, nervousness, weakness, abnormal thinking, agitation, confusion, depersonalization, drowsiness, emotional lability, worsening depression. **EENT:** Mydriasis, rhinitis, visual disturbances, tinnitus. **CV:** Chest pain, hypertension, palpitations, tachycardia. **GI:** Abdominal pain, altered taste, anorexia, constipation, diarrhea, dry mouth, dyspepsia, nausea, vomiting, weight loss. **GU:** Sexual dysfunction, urinary frequency, urinary retention. **Derm:** Ecchymoses, itching, photosensitivity, skin rash. **Neuro:** Paresthesia, twitching. **Misc:** Chills, yawning.

Interactions: Concurrent use with *MAOIs* may result in serious, potentially fatal reactions (wait at least 2 wk after stopping MAO inhibitor before initiating venlafaxine; wait at least 1 wk after stopping venlafaxine before starting MAOIs). Concurrent use with *alcohol* or other *CNS depressants*, including *sedative/hypnotics, antihistamines,* and *opioid analgesics*, in depressed clients is not recommended. ↑ risk of serotonin syndrome with *trazodone, sibutramine,* and *triptans. Lithium* may have ↑ serotonergic effects with venlafaxine; use cautiously in clients receiving venlafaxine. ↑ blood levels and may ↑ effects of *desipramine* and *haloperidol. Cimetidine* may ↑ effects of venlafaxine (may be more pronounced in geriatric clients, those with hepatic or renal impairment, or those with pre-existing hypertension). ***Drug-Natural:*** Concomitant use of *kava-kava, valerian, chamomile,* or hops can ↑ CNS depression. ↑ risk of serotonergic side effects including serotonin syndrome with *St. John's wort* and *SAMe.*

Dosage: PO (Adults): *Tablets:* 50 mg once daily; may ↑ by 50 mg every week up to max dose of 400 mg/day, although additional benefit beyond 50 mg/day was proved only in clinical trials.

Hepatic Impairment: PO (Adults): No dosage adjustment necessary in clients with moderate hepatic impairment, though max daily dose should not exceed 100 mg/day.

Renal Impairment: PO (Adults): *Mild to moderate renal impairment:* No dosage adjustment necessary.

Availability: Brand only

Tablets: 50 mg, 100 mg. COST: **$$$$**

● **Geriatric Considerations:** Caution with CV disease, hypertension, and narrow-angle glaucoma.

- **Pediatric/Adolescent Considerations**: Safety not established. No indication for pediatric use.
- **Clinical Assessments**: Monitor BP before and during Rx. Sustained hypertension may be dose related: ↑ dose or D/C drug. Monitor for suicidality and mood worsening or improvement. Monitor for NMS-like reactions—discontinue drug.

Clinical Tips/Alerts: Be aware of dose-related hypertension. Caution with pre-existing hypertension. Usual and starting dose 50 mg/day. No need to adjust dose unless severe renal/hepatic impairment or end-stage renal disease. However, do not stop abruptly, taper slowly to discontinue. Desvenlafaxine provides once-daily dosing (extended-release formulation) and should not be chewed or crushed, but taken whole.

Dextroamphetamine

(dex-troe-am-**fet**-a-meen) Dexedrine, Dextrostat

Classification: *Therapeutic:* CNS stimulants; *Pharmacological:* Amphetamines; *Schedule II; Pregnancy Category C*

Indications: Narcolepsy. Adjunct management of ADHD. **Off-Label Use:** Exogenous obesity.

Action: Produces CNS stimulation by releasing norepinephrine from nerve endings. Pharmacological effects: CNS and respiratory stimulation, vasoconstriction, mydriasis (pupillary dilation), contraction of urinary bladder sphincter.

Pharmacokinetics: *Absorption:* Well absorbed. *Distribution:* Widely distributed; high concentrations in brain and CSF. Crosses placenta; enters breast milk; potentially embryotoxic. *Metabolism and Excretion:* Some metabolism by liver. Urinary excretion is pH-dependent. Alkaline urine promotes reabsorption and prolongs action.

$T\frac{1}{2}$: 10–12 hr (6.8 hr in children).

TIME/ACTION PROFILE (CNS stimulation)

Route	Onset	Peak	Duration
PO	1–2 hr	3 hr	2–10 hr
PO-ER	Unknown	Unknown	Up to 24 hr

Contraindicated in: *Pregnancy or lactation*. Hyperexcitable states, including hyperthyroidism; psychotic personalities; suicidal or homicidal tendencies; glaucoma; some products contain tartrazine; avoid in clients with known hypersensitivity.

Use Cautiously in: CV disease (sudden death has occurred in children with structural cardiac abnormalities or other serious heart problems); hypertension; diabetes mellitus; history of substance abuse; debilitated clients; continual use may produce psychological dependence or physical addiction.

Adverse Reactions/Side Effects: (CAPITALS indicate life-threatening; underlines indicate most frequent.)

CNS: Hyperactivity, insomnia, restlessness, tremor, depression, dizziness, headache, irritability. **CV:** Palpitations, tachycardia, arrhythmias, hypertension. **GI:** Anorexia, constipation, cramps, diarrhea, dry mouth, metallic taste, nausea, vomiting. **GU:** Erectile dysfunction, ↑ libido. **Derm:** Urticaria. **Misc:** Physical dependence, psychological dependence.

Interactions: ↑ adrenergic effects with other *adrenergics*. Use with *MAOIs* can result in hypertensive crisis. Alkalinizing urine *(sodium bicarbonate, acetazolamide)* prolongs effect. Acidification of urine *(ammonium chloride, large doses of ascorbic acid)* ↓ effect. *Phenothiazines* may ↓ effect of dextroamphetamine. May antagonize response to *antihypertensives*. ↑ risk of CV side effects with *beta blockers or tricyclic antidepressants*. **Drug-Natural:** *St. John's wort* may ↑ serious side effects, concurrent use is not recommended. Use with caffeine-containing herbs *(guarana, tea, coffee)* ↑ stimulant effect. *St. John's wort* may ↑ serious side effects, concurrent use is not recommended.

Dosage: *Attention-Deficit Hyperactivity Disorder:* PO (Adults): 5–40 mg/day in divided doses. Sustained-release capsules should not be used as initial therapy. **PO (Children ≥6 yr):** 5 mg 1–2 times daily, ↑ by 5 mg daily at weekly intervals (maximum: 40 mg/day). Sustained-release capsules should not be used as initial therapy. **PO (Children 3–5 yr):** 2.5 mg/day, ↑ by 2.5 mg daily at weekly intervals (maximum: 40 mg/day). *Narcolepsy:* PO (Adults): 5–60 mg/day single dose or in divided doses. Sustained-release capsules should not be used as initial therapy. **PO (Children ≥12 yr):** 10 mg/day, ↑ by 10 mg/day at weekly intervals until response is obtained 60 mg is reached. **PO (Children 6–12 yr):** 5 mg/day, ↑ by 5 mg/day at weekly intervals until response obtained or 60 mg reached. *Exogenous obesity:* PO (Adults and Children >12 yr): 5–30 mg/day in divided doses of 5–10 mg given 30–60 min before meals.

Availability (generic available)

Tablets: 5 mg. **Sustained-release capsules:** 5 mg, 10 mg, 15 mg.

DRUGS D-G

Diazepam

(dye-**az**-e-pam) Valium, Diastat, Apo-Diazepam, Diazemuls, Novodipam, PMS-Diazepam, Vivol

Classification: *Therapeutic:* Antianxiety agents, anticonvulsants, sedatives/hypnotics, skeletal muscle relaxants (centrally acting)
Pharmacological: Benzodiazepines; *Schedule IV; Pregnancy Category D*

Indications: Adjunct in management of: Anxiety disorder, athetosis, anxiety relief before cardioversion (injection), Stiffman syndrome, preoperative sedation, conscious sedation (provides light anesthesia and anterograde amnesia); Treatment of status epilepticus/uncontrolled seizures (injection), Skeletal muscle relaxant, Management of symptoms of alcohol withdrawal. **Off-Label Use:** Anxiety associated with acute myocardial infarction, insomnia.

Action: Depresses CNS, probably by potentiating GABA, an inhibitory neurotransmitter. Produces skeletal muscle relaxation by inhibiting spinal polysynaptic afferent pathways. Has anticonvulsant properties due to enhanced presynaptic inhibition.

Pharmacokinetics: *Absorption:* Rapidly absorbed from GI tract. Absorption from IM sites may be slow and unpredictable. Well absorbed (90%) from rectal mucosa.
Distribution: Widely distributed. Crosses blood–brain barrier. Crosses placenta, enters breast milk.
Metabolism and Excretion: Highly metabolized by liver. Some products of metabolism are active as CNS depressants.
T ½: Neonates: 50–95 hr; infants 1 month–2 yr: 40–50 hr; children 2–12 yr: 15–21 hr; children 12–16 yr: 18–20 hr; adults: 20–50 hr (up to 100 hr for metabolites).

● **Geriatric Considerations:** On Beers list of drugs; elderly should avoid. May ↑ hypertension, cause angina, MI.
● **Pediatric/Adolescent Considerations:** Caution with CV disease, sudden death has occurred. Monitor weight for weight loss.
● **Substance Abuse Considerations:** High dependence and potential for abuse.
● **Clinical Assessments:** Monitor BP, pulse, and respiration before and after Rx. Monitor attention and impulse control.

[**Clinical Tips/Alerts:** Use lowest effective dose, and be aware of dependence and fairly rapid tolerance to drug. ↑ slowly if at all. Rebound mood lability and hyperactivity can occur after medication wears off.]

TIME/ACTION PROFILE (sedation)

Route	Onset	Peak	Duration
PO	30–60 min	1–2 hr	Up to 24 hr
IM	Within 20 min	0.5–1.5 hr	Unknown
IV	1–5 min	15–30 min	15–60 min*
Rectal	2–10 min	1–2 hr	4–12 hr

*In status epilepticus, anticonvulsant duration is 15–20 min

Contraindicated in: *Pregnancy or lactation.* Hypersensitivity; cross-sensitivity with other benzodiazepines may occur; comatose clients; pre-existing CNS depression; uncontrolled severe pain; angle-closure glaucoma;; some products contain alcohol, propylene glycol, or tartrazine and should be avoided in clients with known hyper sensitivity or intolerance. *Pregnancy:* ↑ risk of congenital malformations. *Lactation:* Discontinue drug or bottle feed.

Use Cautiously in: Hepatic dysfunction; severe renal impairment; severe pulmonary impairment; history of suicide attempt or drug dependence; debilitated clients (dose reduction required); clients with low albumin.

Adverse Reactions/Side Effects: (CAPITALS indicate life-threatening; underlines indicate most frequent.)

CNS: Dizziness, drowsiness, lethargy, depression, hangover, ataxia, slurred speech, headache, paradoxical excitation. **EENT:** Blurred vision. **Resp:** Respiratory depression. **CV:** Hypotension (IV only). **GI:** Constipation, diarrhea (may be caused by propylene glycol content in oral solution), nausea, vomiting, weight gain. **Derm:** Rashes. **Local:** Pain (IM), phlebitis (IV), venous thrombosis. **Misc:** Physical dependence, psychological dependence, tolerance.

Interactions: *Alcohol, antidepressants, antihistamines,* and *opioid analgesics—* concurrent use results in additive CNS depression. *Cimetidine, hormonal contraceptives, disulfiram, fluoxetine, isoniazid, ketoconazole, metoprolol, propoxyphene, propranolol, or valproic acid* may ↓ metabolism of diazepam, enhancing its actions. May ↓ efficacy of *levodopa. Rifampin* or *barbiturates* may ↑ metabolism and ↓ effectiveness of diazepam. Sedative effects may be ↓ by *theophylline.* Concurrent use of *ritonavir* is not recommended. *Drug-Natural:* Concomitant use of *kava, valerian,* or *chamomile* can ↑ CNS depression.

Dosage: *Antianxiety: PO (Adults):* 2–10 mg 2–4 times daily.

IM, IV (Adults): 2–10 mg, may repeat in 3–4 hrs as needed.

PO (Children >1 mo): 0.12–0.8 mg/kg/day 3–4 times daily.

IM, IV (Children >1 mo): 0.04–0.3 mg/kg/dose every 2–4 hr to a maximum of 0.6 mg/kg within an 8-hr period if necessary.

Alcohol Withdrawal: PO (Adults): 10 mg 3–4 times in first 24 hr, ↓ to 5 mg 3–4 times daily.

IM, IV (Adults): 10 mg initially, then 5–10 mg in 3–4 hr as needed; larger or more frequent doses have been used.

Psychoneurotic Reactions: IM, IV (Adults): 2–10 mg, may be repeated in 3–4 hr.

Availability (generic available)

Tablets: 2 mg, 5 mg, 10 mg. COST: *Generic* **$.** **Oral solution:** 5 mg/mL (Intensol), 1 mg/mL. **Solution for injection:** 5 mg/mL (contains 10% alcohol and 40% propylene glycol). **Rectal gel delivery system:** 2.5 mg, 10 mg, 20 mg.

● **Geriatric Considerations:** On Beers list with ↑ risk for falls (long-acting benzodiazepine) and sedation. Use short-acting or ↓ dose.

● **Pediatric/Adolescent Considerations:** Fatal gasping syndrome in neonates, with injection. Neonates accumulate metabolites. Use with caution in children/adolescents. Monitor for sedation, dizziness, ataxia, abuse (esp. with adolescents).

● **Substance Abuse Considerations:** Dependence and tolerance with long-term use.

● **Clinical Assessments:** Monitor BP, pulse, and respirations before and during Rx, esp. IV. Assess if Rx necessary periodically.

Clinical Tips/Alerts: Used for alcohol withdrawal and sleep disorders (night terrors). Use lowest effective dose and taper slowly if discontinuing. Consider 1 month of tapering for each year of dependence.

Donepezil

(doe-**nep**-i-zill) Aricept, Aricept ODT

Classification: *Therapeutic:* Anti-Alzheimer's agents
Pharmacological: Cholinergics (cholinesterase inhibitors); *Pregnancy Category C*

Indications: Mild to moderate dementia associated with Alzheimer's disease.

Action: Inhibits acetylcholinesterase, thus improving cholinergic function by making more acetylcholine available.

Pharmacokinetics: *Absorption:* Well absorbed after oral administration. *Distribution:* Unknown.

Metabolism and Excretion: Partially metabolized by liver (CYP2D6 and CYP3A4 enyzmes) and partially excreted by kidneys (17% unchanged). Two metabolites pharmacologically active.

Protein Binding: 96%.

T $^1/_2$: 70 hr.

TIME/ACTION PROFILE (improvement in symptoms)

Route	Onset	Peak	Duration
PO	Unknown	Several weeks	6 wk*

*Return to baseline after discontinuation

Contraindicated in: Hypersensitivity to donepezil or piperidine derivatives.

Use Cautiously in: Clients with underlying cardiac disease, esp. sick sinus syndrome or supraventricular conduction defects; clients with a history of ulcer disease or those currently taking NSAIDs; clients with a history of seizures; clients with a history of asthma or obstructive pulmonary disease. *Pregnancy/Lactation:* Safety not established; assumed to be secreted in breast milk. Discontinue drug or bottle-feed.

Adverse Reactions/Side Effects: (CAPITALS indicate life-threatening; underlines indicate most frequent.)

CNS: Headache, abnormal dreams, depression, dizziness, drowsiness, fatigue, insomnia, syncope, sedation (unusual). **CV:** Atrial fibrillation, hypertension, hypotension, vasodilation. **GI:** Diarrhea, nausea, anorexia, vomiting, weight gain (unusual). **GU:** Frequent urination. **Derm:** Ecchymoses. **Metab:** Hot flashes, weight loss. **MS:** Arthritis, muscle cramps.

Interactions: Exaggerates muscle relaxation from *succinylcholine.* Interferes with action of *anticholinergics.* ↑ Cholinergic effects of *bethanechol.* May ↑ risk of GI bleeding from *NSAIDs. Quinidine* and *ketoconazole* ↓ metabolism of donepezil. *Rifampin, carbamazepine, dexamethasone, phenobarbital,* and *phenytoin* induce enzymes that metabolize donepezil and may ↓ its effects. ***Drug-Natural:*** *Jimson weed* and *scopolia* may antagonize cholinergic effects.

Donepezil/Doxepin

Dosage: Mild to Moderate Alzheimer's Disease: PO (Adults): 5 mg once daily; after 4–6 wk may ↑ to 10 mg once daily (dose should not exceed 5 mg/day in frail, elderly females).

Severe Alzheimer's Disease: PO (Adults): 10 mg once daily (dose should not exceed 10 mg/day).

Availability: Brand only

Tablets: 5 mg, 10 mg. COST: **$$$$ Orally disintegrating tablets:** 5 mg, 10 mg.
COST: **$$$**

- **Geriatric Considerations:** Elderly may require lower doses.
- **Pediatric/Adolescent Considerations:** Safety not established. No indications although studies have been conducted to evaluate efficacy in treatment of ADHD.
- **Clinical Assessments:** Evaluate cognitive baseline and cognitive decline through Mini-Mental State Exam and clock drawing tests (which involves simultaneous cognitive, motor, and perceptual functions). These are screening tools, and further diagnostic tests may be needed. Evaluate for cardiac disease; monitor pulse and heart rate. Also Geriatric Depression Scale or other depression scale. Be cognizant of *pseudodementia* (depression that appears to be dementia because of cognitive impairments). A client may exhibit both dementia and depression, which need treatment.

Clinical Tips/Alerts: May also need other treatments for behavioral problems or depression, such as mood stabilizers or antidepressants. There is an ↑ chance of mortality with use of atypical/conventional antipsychotics in the elderly with dementia-related psychosis. Family members are good indicators of observed improvement or decline.

Doxepin

(**dox**-e-pin) Sinequan, Zonalon, *Triadapin*

Classification: *Therapeutic:* Antianxiety agents, antidepressants, antihistamines (topical); *Pharmacological:* Tricyclic antidepressants; *Pregnancy Category C*

Indications: PO: Depression. **Off-Label Use: PO:** Chronic pain syndromes; anxiety, insomnia.

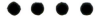

Action: PO: Prevents reuptake of norepinephrine and serotonin by presynaptic neurons; resultant accumulation of neurotransmitters potentiates their activity. Also possesses significant anticholinergic properties. **Topical:** Antipruritic action due to antihistaminic properties.

Pharmacokinetics: *Absorption:* Well absorbed from GI tract, although much is metabolized on first pass through liver. Some systemic absorption follows topical application.

Distribution: Widely distributed. Enters breast milk; probably crosses the placenta.

Metabolism and Excretion: Metabolized by the liver. Some conversion to active anti-depressant compound. May re-enter gastric juice via secretion from enterohepatic circulation, where more absorption may occur.

T $^1/_2$: 8–25 hr.

TIME/ACTION PROFILE (antidepressant activity)

Route	Onset	Peak	Duration
PO	2–3 wk	Up to 6 wk	Days-weeks

Contraindicated in: Hypersensitivity; some products contain bisulfites and should be avoided in clients with known intolerance; untreated angle-closure glaucoma; period immediately after myocardial infarction; history of QTc prolongation, heart failure, cardiac arrhythmia.

Use Cautiously in: Pre-existing CV disease ($\uparrow$ risk of adverse reactions); prostat-ic enlargement (more susceptible to urinary retention); seizures. *Pregnancy:* Use during pregnancy only if potential maternal benefit outweighs risks to fetus; use during *lactation* may result in neonatal sedation. Recommend discontinue drug or bottle-feed.

Adverse Reactions/Side Effects: (CAPITALS indicate life-threatening; underlines indicate most frequent.)

CNS: Fatigue, sedation, agitation, confusion, hallucinations. **EENT:** Blurred vision, $\uparrow$ intraocular pressure. **CV:** Hypotension, arrhythmias, ECG abnormalities. **GI:** Constipation, dry mouth, hepatitis, $\uparrow$ appetite, weight gain, nausea, paralytic ileus. **GU:** Urinary retention, $\downarrow$ libido. **Derm:** Photosensitivity, rashes. **Hemat:** Blood dyscrasias. **Misc:** Hypersensitivity reactions.

Interactions: *Applies to topical and oral use:* Doxepin metabolized in liver by cytochrome P450 2D6 enzyme and its action may be affected by drugs that compete for metabolism by this enzyme, including other antidepressants, phenothiazines, carbamazepine, class 1C antiarrhythmics (propafenone, flecainide); when used concurrently, dosage ↓ of one or the other or both may be necessary. Concurrent use of other drugs that inhibit activity of the enzyme, including cimetidine, quinidine, amiodarone, and ritonavir, may result in ↑ effects of doxepin. May cause hypotension, tachycardia, and potentially fatal reactions when used with MAOIs (avoid concurrent use; discontinue MAOIs 2 wk before doxepin). Concurrent use with SSRI antidepressants may result in ↑ toxicity and should be avoided (fluoxetine should be stopped 5 wk before). Concurrent use with clonidine may result ↓ hypertensive crisis and should be avoided. Concurrent use with levodopa or hypertension. Blood levodopa may result in delayed ↓ absorption of levodopa or hypertension. Blood levels and effects may be ↓ by rifamycins. ↑ CNS depression with other CNS depressants including alcohol, antihistamines, clonidine, opioid analgesics, and sedatives/hypnotics. Barbiturates may alter blood levels and effects. *Adrenergic and anticholinergic side effects may be ↑ with other agents having these properties.* Phenothiazines or hormonal contraceptives ↑ levels and may cause toxicity. Smoking may ↑ metabolism and alter effects. *Drug-Natural:* Concomitant use of kava, valerian, or chamomile can ↑ CNS depression. ↑ Anticholinergic effects with jimson weed and scopolia.

Dosage: PO (Adults): *Antidepressant/anti-anxiety:* 25 mg 3 times daily, may be ↑ as needed (up to 150 mg/day for outpatients or 300 mg/day for inpatients; some clients may require only 25–50 mg/day). Once stabilized, entire daily dose may be given at bedtime. **PO (Geriatric Clients):** *Antidepressant:* 25–50 mg/day initially, may be ↑ as needed.

Availability (generic available)

Capsules: 10 mg, 25 mg, 50 mg, 75 mg, 100 mg, 150 mg. **Oral concentrate:** 10 mg/mL. **Topical cream:** 5%. COST: $

● **Geriatric Considerations:** As with all tricyclics, caution with pre-existing CV disease, BPH, urinary retention; ↑ chance of falls due to sedation, anticholinergic effects, and hypotension. On Beers list of inappropriate drugs for elderly. Reduce initial dose.

● **Pediatric/Adolescent Considerations:** Safety not established in children <12 yr). May ↑ risk of suicide attempt/ideation esp. during early treatment or dose adjustment; risk may be greater in children or adolescents. Monitor face-to-face early in Rx and during dose adjustments.

● **Clinical Assessments:** History CV disease or high doses, ECG before starting Rx and periodically. Also monitor BP, pulse before and after Rx. Monitor weight and BMI before and during Rx as weight gain is common (*see BMI/Metabolic Syndrome, Tools Tab*); also FBS, cholesterol, and electrolytes. Assess elderly for risk of falls. Assess for depression using rating scales before and during Rx.

Clinical Tips/Alerts: All clients need to be monitored for possibility of suicidality once treatment started; clients should be asked directly if they are feeling suicidal or considering suicide. ↑ Doses at bedtime. Deaths have occurred from overdosage; avoid alcohol.

Duloxetine

(do-**lox**-e-teen) Cymbalta

Classification: *Therapeutic:* Antidepressants; *Pharmacological:* Selective serotonin norepinephrine reuptake inhibitors; *Pregnancy Category C*

Indications: Major depressive disorder. Management of diabetic peripheral neuropathic pain. Generalized anxiety disorder: diabetic peripheral neuropathic pain (DPNP). **Off-Label Use:** Stress urinary incontinence. Neuropathic pain/chronic pain. Fibromyalgia. GAD.

Action: Inhibits serotonin and norepinephrine reuptake in CNS. Both antidepressant and pain inhibition are mediated centrally. Neuropathic pain. ↓ Symptoms of anxiety.

Pharmacokinetics: *Absorption:* Well absorbed following oral administration. *Distribution:* Unknown. *Metabolism and Excretion:* Mostly metabolized, primarily by CYP2D6 and CYP1A2 enzyme pathways.

Protein Binding: Highly (>90%) protein-bound.

T $\frac{1}{2}$: 12 hr.

TIME/ACTION PROFILE (blood levels)

Route	Onset	Peak	Duration
PO	Unknown	6 hr	12 hr

Contraindicated in: Hypersensitivity; concurrent MAOI therapy; uncontrolled angle-closure glaucoma; end-stage renal disease; chronic hepatic impairment or substantial alcohol use (↑ risk of hepatitis). *Lactation:* May enter breast milk; discontinue or bottle-feed.

Use Cautiously in: History of suicide attempt or ideation; history of mania (may activate mania/hypomania); concurrent use of other centrally acting drugs (↑ risk of adverse reactions); history of seizure disorder; controlled angle-closure glaucoma; diabetic clients and those with renal impairment (consider lower initial dose with gradual increase). *Pregnancy:* Use during third trimester may result in neonatal serotonin syndrome requiring prolonged hospitalization and respiratory and nutritional support.

Adverse Reactions/Side Effects: (CAPITALS indicate life-threatening; underlines indicate most frequent.)

CNS: SEIZURES, fatigue, drowsiness, insomnia, activation of mania, dizziness, nightmares. **EENT:** Blurred vision, ↑ intraocular pressure. **CV:** ↑ BP. **GI:** ↑ Appetite, constipation, dry mouth, nausea, diarrhea, ↑ liver enzymes, gastritis, hepatitis, vomiting. **GU:** Dysuria, abnormal orgasm, erectile dysfunction, ↑ libido, urinary hesitation. **Derm:** Sweating, pruritus, rash. **Neuro:** Tremor.

Interactions: Concurrent use with MAOIs may result in serious, potentially fatal reactions (do not use within 14 days of discontinuing MAOI; wait at least 5 days after stopping duloxetine to start MAOI). ↑ Risk of hepatotoxicity with chronic alcohol abuse. Drugs that affect serotonergic neurotransmitter systems, including linezolid, tramadol, and triptans ↑ risk of serotonin syndrome. *Drugs that inhibit CYP1A2,* including fluvoxamine and some fluoroquinolones ↑ levels of duloxetine and should be avoided. *Drugs that inhibit CYP2D6,* including paroxetine, fluoxetine, and quinidine, ↑ levels of duloxetine and may ↑ risk of adverse reactions. Duloxetine also inhibits CYP2D6 and may ↑ levels of drugs metabolized by CYP2D6, including *tricyclic antidepressants, phenothiazines,* and *class 1C antiarrhythmics (propafenone* and *flecainide);* concurrent use should be undertaken with caution. ↑ Risk of serious arrhythmias with thioridazine; avoid concurrent use. *Drug-Natural:* Use with *St. John's wort* ↑ serotonin syndrome.

Dosage: PO (Adults): *Antidepressant:* 20–30 mg twice daily, for neuropathic pain or generalized anxiety disorder: 60 mg once daily; may ↑ up to 120 mg daily. **Renal Impairment: PO (Adults):** Start with lower dose and ↑ gradually.

Availability
Capsules: 20 mg, 30 mg, 60 mg. COST: $$$$

- **Geriatric Considerations:** Elderly may require lower doses.
- **Pediatric/Adolescent Considerations**: May ↑ risk of suicide attempt/ ideation esp. during early treatment or dose adjustment; risk may be greater in children or adolescents (safe use in children/adolescents not established).
- **Clinical Assessments:** Monitor for mood improvement and suicidality throughout Rx; assess depression severity using a depression rating scale. Monitor BP before and during Rx; ↑ BP dose-related and may require dose reduction or alternate Rx.

Clinical Tips/Alerts: Concurrent use with MAOI potentially fatal. Do not use within 14 days of discontinuing MAOI. Wait at least 5 days after stopping duloxetine to start MAOI. Always need to be vigilant for possibility of suicide even with (or maybe especially with) mood improvement and physical activity.

Escitalopram

(ess-sit-**al**-o-pram) Lexapro

Classification: *Therapeutic:* Antidepressants; *Pharmacological:* SSRIs; *Pregnancy Category C*

Indications: Major depressive disorder. Major depressive disorder (acute and maintenance) in adolescents (12–17 yr). GAD. **Off-Label Use:** Panic disorder. OCD. Post-traumatic stress disorder (PTSD). Social anxiety discorder (social phobia). PMDD.

Action: Selectively inhibits reuptake of serotonin in the CNS.

Pharmacokinetics: *Absorption:* 80% absorbed following oral administration. *Distribution:* Enters breast milk.

Metabolism and Excretion: Mostly metabolized by liver (primarily CYP3A4 and CYP2C19 isoenzymes); 7% excreted unchanged by kidneys.

T $^1/_2$: ↑ in geriatric clients and clients with hepatic impairment.

TIME/ACTION PROFILE (antidepressant effect)

Route	Onset	Peak	Duration
PO	Within 1–4 wk	Unknown	Unknown

Contraindicated in: Hypersensitivity; concurrent MAOIs; concurrent citalopram.

Use Cautiously in: History of mania (may activate mania/hypomania); history of seizures; clients at risk for suicide; hepatic impairment (dose reduction recommended); severe renal impairment. **Pregnancy:** Neonates exposed to SSRI in third trimester may develop drug discontinuation syndrome, including respiratory distress, feeding difficulty, and irritability. Weigh risks and benefits. **Lactation:** May cause adverse effects in infant; risk/benefit should be considered.

Adverse Reactions/Side Effects: (CAPITALS indicate life-threatening; underlines indicate most frequent.)

CNS: Insomnia, dizziness, drowsiness, fatigue. **GI:** Diarrhea, nausea, abdominal pain, constipation, dry mouth, indigestion. **GU:** Anorgasmia, ↓ libido, ejaculatory delay, erectile dysfunction. **Derm:** ↑ Sweating. **Endo:** Syndrome on inappropriate secretion of antidiuretic hormone (SIADH). **F and E:** Hyponatremia. **Metab:** ↑ Appetite.

Interactions: May cause serious, potentially fatal reactions when used with MAOIs; allow at least 14 days between escitalopram and MAOIs. Use cautiously with other centrally acting drugs (including alcohol, antihistamines, opioid analgesics, and sedatives/hypnotics; concurrent use with alcohol is not recommended). Concurrent use with sumatriptan or other 5-HT₃ agonist vascular headache suppressants may result in weakness, hyperreflexia, and incoordination. Cimetidine ↑ blood levels of escitalopram. Serotonergic effects may be ↑ by lithium (concurrent use should be carefully monitored). Carbamazepine may ↑ blood levels. May ↑ blood levels of metoprolol. Concurrent use with tricyclic antidepressants should be undertaken with caution because of altered pharmacokinetics. **Drug-Natural:** ↑ Risk of serotonin syndrome with St. John's wort and SAMe.

Dosage: PO (Adults): 10 mg once daily, may be ↑ to 20 mg once daily after 1 wk. **Hepatic Impairment: PO (Adults):** 10 mg once daily. **PO (Geriatric Clients):** 10 mg once daily. **PO (Adolescents 12–17 yr):** 10 mg once daily; may ↑ to 20 mg once daily after 3 weeks.

Availability

Tablets: 5 mg, 10 mg, 20 mg. COST: **$$$$. Oral solution (peppermint):** 1 mg/mL in 240-mL bottles. COST: **$$.**

● **Geriatric Considerations:** Reduce dose esp. with hepatic impairment.
● **Pediatric/Adolescent Considerations:** May ↑ risk of suicide attempt/ideation esp. during early treatment or dose adjustment in children/adolescents (off label for pediatric use). Children require face-to-face monitoring early on and during dosage adjustments.

● **Clinical Assessments:** Monitor all clients for mood improvement and for suicidality. Assess for sexual dysfunction (erectile dysfunction, anorgasmia, ↓ sexual desire).

[**Clinical Tips/Alerts:** Use with MAOIs potentially fatal (see Interactions). If anorgasmia very problematic in women, bupropion may be considered.]

Eszopiclone

(es-**zop**-i-klone) Lunesta

Classification: *Therapeutic:* Sedatives/hypnotics; *Pharmacological:* Cyclopyrrolones; *Schedule IV; Pregnancy Category C*

Indications: Insomnia, sleep latency, and maintenance.

Action: Interacts with GABA-receptor complexes; not a benzodiazepine.

Pharmacokinetics: *Absorption:* Rapidly absorbed after oral administration. *Distribution:* Unknown. *Metabolism and Excretion:* Extensively metabolized by liver (CYP3A4 and CYP2E1 enzyme systems); metabolites excreted renally, <10% excreted unchanged in urine.

T $\frac{1}{2}$: 6 hr.

TIME/ACTION PROFILE (blood levels)

Route	Onset	Peak	Duration
PO	Rapid	1 hr	6 hr

Contraindicated in: No known contraindications.

Use Cautiously in: Geriatric/debilitated clients (may have ↓ metabolism or ↑ sensitivity; use lower initial dose); conditions that may alter metabolic or hemodynamic function; severe hepatic impairment (use lower initial dose).

Pregnancy/Lactation: Safety not established; use only if maternal benefit justifies fetal risk.

Adverse Reactions/Side Effects (CAPITALS indicate life-threatening; underlines indicate most frequent.)

CNS: Abnormal thinking, behavior changes, depression, hallucinations, headache, sleep driving. **CV:** Chest pain, peripheral edema. **GI:** Dry mouth, unpleasant taste. **Derm:** Rash.

Interactions: ↑ Risk of CNS depression with other CNS depressants including antihistamines, antidepressants, opioids, sedatives/hypnotics, and antipsychotics. ↑ Levels and risk of CNS depression with drugs that inhibit CYP3A4 enzyme system, including ketoconazole, itraconazole, clarithromycin, nefazodone, ritonavir, and nelfinavir. Levels and effectiveness may be ↑ by drugs that induce CYP3A4 enzyme system, including rifampicin.

Dosage: PO (Adults): 2 mg immediately before bedtime, may be raised to 3 mg if needed (3 mg dose more effective for sleep maintenance); Geriatric clients: 1 mg immediately before bedtime for clients with difficulty falling asleep, 2 mg for clients who have difficulty staying asleep.

Hepatic Impairment: PO (Adults): Severe hepatic impairment: 1 mg immediately before bedtime. **PO (Adults receiving concurrent CYP3A4 inhibitors):** 1 mg immediately before bedtime, may be raised to 2 mg if needed.

Availability: Brand only
Tablets: 1 mg, 2 mg, 3 mg. COST: $$$
- **Geriatric Considerations:** Use lower initial dose (start 1 mg); may have ↓ sensitivity and ↑ metabolism.
- **Pediatric/Adolescent Considerations:** Children <18 yr (safety not established).
- **Substance Abuse Considerations:** Prolonged use may lead to dependence.
- **Clinical Assessments:** Assess sleep patterns before and during Rx. Monitor for substance dependence/abuse.

Clinical Tips/Alerts: Clients have been known to perform activities (cook/eat/drive) while asleep (complex sleep-related behaviors) and serious allergic reactions have happened (swelling of tongue/throat, difficulty breathing) requiring emergency care. If angioedema develops, seek emergency treatment, and do not use drug again. Take immediately before bed as onset is rapid.

Fluoxetine

(floo-ox-uh-teen) Prozac, Prozac Weekly, Sarafem

Classification: *Therapeutic:* antidepressants; *Pharmacological:* SSRIs; *Pregnancy Category C*

Indications: Various forms of depression, including depression in children ages 8–17 yr; OCD, including children ages 7–17. Bulimia nervosa. Panic disorder.

Sarafem: Management of PMDD. **Off-Label Use:** Anorexia nervosa: ADHD, diabetic neuropathy, fibromyalgia, obesity, Raynaud's phenomenon, social anxiety disorder (social phobia), PTSD.

Action: Selectively inhibits reuptake of serotonin in CNS.

Pharmacokinetics: *Absorption:* Well absorbed after oral administration. *Distribution:* Crosses blood-brain barrier.

Metabolism and Excretion: Converted by liver to norfluoxetine, another antidepressant compound; fluoxetine and norfluoxetine are mostly metabolized by the liver; 12% excreted by kidneys as unchanged fluoxetine, 7% as unchanged norfluoxetine.

Protein Binding: 94.5%.

T $^1/_2$: 1–3 days (norfluoxetine 5–7 days).

TIME/ACTION PROFILE (antidepressant activity)

Route	Onset	Peak	Duration
PO	1–4 wk	Unknown	2 wk

Contraindicated in: Hypersensitivity; concurrent use or use within 14 days of discontinuing MAOIs (fluoxetine should be discontinued 5 wk before MAO therapy is initiated).

Use Cautiously in: Severe hepatic or renal impairment (lower/less frequent dose may be necessary); history of seizures; debilitated clients (↑ risk of seizures); diabetes mellitus; clients with concurrent chronic illness or multiple drug therapy (dose adjustments may be necessary); clients with impaired hepatic function (lower doses/↑ dosing interval may be necessary); may ↑ risk of suicide attempt/ideation, esp. during early treatment or dose adjustment. *Pregnancy:* Use during third trimester may result in neonatal serotonin syndrome requiring prolonged hospitalization and respiratory and nutritional support. May cause sedation in infant. *Lactation:* May cause sedation in infant; discontinue drug or bottle-feed.

Adverse Reactions/Side Effects: (CAPITALS indicate life-threatening; underlines indicate most frequent.)

CNS: SEIZURES, anxiety, drowsiness, headache, insomnia, nervousness, abnormal dreams, dizziness, fatigue, hypomania, mania, weakness. **EENT:** Stuffy nose, visual disturbances. **Resp:** Cough. **CV:** Chest pain, palpitations. **GI:** Diarrhea, abdominal pain, abnormal taste, anorexia, constipation, dry mouth, dyspepsia, nausea, vomiting, weight loss. **GU:** Sexual dysfunction, urinary frequency. **Derm:** Excessive sweating, pruritus, erythema nodosum, flushing, rashes. **Endo:** Dysmenorrhea. **MS:** Arthralgia, back pain, myalgia. **Neuro:** Tremor. **Misc:** Allergic reactions, fever, flu-like syndrome, hot flashes, sensitivity reaction.

Interactions: Discontinue use of MAOIs for 14 days before fluoxetine therapy; combined therapy may result in confusion, agitation, seizures, hypertension, and hyperpyrexia (serotonin syndrome). Fluoxetine should be discontinued for at least 5 wk before MAOI therapy is initiated. Inhibits activity of cytochrome P450 2D6 enzyme in liver and ↑ effects of drugs metabolized by this enzyme system. *Medications that inhibit the P450 enzyme system* (including *ritonavir, saquinavir,* and *efavirenz)* may ↑ risk of developing the serotonin syndrome. For concurrent use with ritonavir, ↑ fluoxetine dose by 70%; if initiating fluoxetine, start with 10 mg/day dose. ↑ Metabolism and ↑ effects of alprazolam (↑ alprazolam dose by 50%). CNS depression with alcohol, antihistamines, other antidepressants, opioid analgesics, or sedatives/hypnotics. ↑ Risk of side effects and adverse reactions with other antidepressants, tryptophan, risperidone, or phenothiazines. May ↑ effectiveness/risk of toxicity from carbamazepine, clozapine, digoxin, haloperidol, phenytoin, lithium, or warfarin. May ↑ the effects of buspirone. Cyproheptadine may ↓ or reverse effects of fluoxetine. May ↑ sensitivity to adrenergics and ↑ the risk of serotonin syndrome. May alter the activity of other drugs that are highly bound to plasma proteins. **Drug-Natural:** ↑ Risk of serotonin syndrome with *St. John's wort* and SAME.

Dosage: PO (Adults): Depression, OCD: 20 mg/day in the morning. After several weeks, may ↑ by 20 mg/day at weekly intervals. Doses greater than 20 mg/day should be given in two divided doses, in the morning and at noon (not to exceed 80 mg/day). Clients who have been stabilized on the 20-mg/day dose may be switched to delayed-release capsules (Prozac Weekly) at dose of 90 mg weekly, initiated 7 days after the last 20-mg dose. **Panic disorder:** 10 mg/day initially, may ↑ after 1 week to 20 mg/day (usual dose is 20 mg, but may be ↑ as needed/tolerated up to 60 mg/day). **Bulimia nervosa:** 60 mg/day (may need to titrate up to dosage over several days). **PMDD:** 20 mg/day (not to exceed 80 mg/day) *or* 20 mg/day starting 14 days before expected onset of menses, continued through first full day of menstruation, repeated with each cycle.
PO (Geriatric Clients): Depression: 10 mg/day in the morning initially, may be ↑ (not to exceed 60 mg/day).

PO (Children 7–17 yr): *Adolescents and higher-weight children:* 10 mg/day may be ↑ after 2 wk to 20 mg/day; additional increases may be made after several more weeks (range 20–60 mg/day); *lower-weight children:* 10 mg/day initially, may be ↑ after several more weeks (range 20–30 mg/day).

Availability (generic available)

Tablets: 10 mg, 20 mg. COST: *Generic* **$**. **Capsules:** 10 mg, 20 mg, 40 mg. COST: *Generic* **$**. **Delayed-release capsules (Prozac Weekly):** 90 mg. COST: **$$**. Oral solution (mint flavor): 20 mg/5 mL. COST: *Generic* **$$**. *In combination with:* olanzapine (Symbyax). (See olanzapine, Drug Tab N-Q.)

- **Geriatric Considerations:** ↑ Risk for agitation and sleep disturbances; on Beers list. Because of long half-life consider lower dosing or dosing every other day; not to exceed 60 mg/day.
- **Pediatric/Adolescent Considerations:** Approved for depression and OCD in children and adolescents; ↑ risk for suicide in children; monitor face-to-face for suicidal thoughts early on and during dosage adjustments. Monitor for ↑ agitation and excitability (disinhibition). Safety not established <7 yr.
- **Clinical Assessments:** Monitor for improvement of mood, ↑ in anxiety or insomnia. Monitor closely for suicidality. Weigh client before Rx, and observe for notable weight loss.

> **Clinical Tips/Alerts:** Discontinue fluoxetine at least 5 wk before starting MAOIs; discontinue MAOIs at least 2 wk before starting fluoxetine because of risk of serotonin syndrome. Consider Prozac Weekly after client is stabilized. Prozac Weekly esp. useful for adolescents who do not like to take medication. OCD usually requires larger doses (divided: morning and noon) per day.

Fluphenazine

(floo-**fen**-a-zeen) Prolixin, Prolixin Decanoate, *Apo-Fluphenazine, Modecate Concentrate, PMS-Fluphenazine*

Classification: *Therapeutic:* Antipsychotics; *Pharmacological:* Phenothiazines; *Pregnancy Category C*

Indications: Acute and chronic psychoses.

Action: Alters the effects of dopamine in CNS. Anticholinergic and alpha-adrenergic blocking activity.

Pharmacokinetics: *Absorption:* Well absorbed after PO/IM administration.

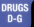

Decanoate salt in sesame oil has delayed onset and prolonged action because of delayed release from oil vehicle and subsequent delayed release from fatty tissues.

Distribution: Widely distributed. Crosses blood-brain barrier. Crosses placenta; enters breast milk.

Metabolism and Excretion: Highly metabolized by liver; undergoes enterohepatic recirculation.

Protein Binding: ≥90%.

T $\frac{1}{2}$: Fluphenazine hydrochloride: 33 hr; fluphenazine decanoate: 6.8–9.6 days.

TIME/ACTION PROFILE (antipsychotic activity)

Route	Onset	Peak	Duration
PO hydrochloride	1 hr	Unknown	6–8 hr
IM decanoate	24–72 hr	48–96 hr	≥4 wk

Contraindicated in: Hypersensitivity; cross-sensitivity with other phenothiazines may exist; subcortical brain damage; severe CNS depression; coma; bone marrow depression; liver disease; hypersensitivity to sesame oil (decanoate salt); some products contain alcohol or tartrazine and should be avoided in clients with known intolerance; concurrent use of drugs that prolong QT interval.

Use Cautiously in: CV disease: Parkinson's disease; angle-closure glaucoma; myasthenia gravis; prostatic hypertrophy; seizure disorders; debilitated clients. **Lactation:** Enters breast milk, discontinue or bottle-feed. **Pregnancy:** Safety not established.

Adverse Reactions/Side Effects: (CAPITALS indicate life-threatening; underlines indicate most frequent.)
CNS: NEUROLEPTIC MALIGNANT SYNDROME, extrapyramidal reactions, sedation, tardive dyskinesia. **EENT:** Blurred vision, dry eyes. **CV:** Hypertension, hypotension, tachycardia. **GI:** Anorexia, constipation, drug-induced hepatitis, dry mouth, ileus, nausea, weight gain. **GU:** Urinary retention. **Derm:** Photosensitivity, pigment changes, rashes. **Endo:** Galactorrhea. **Hemat:** AGRANULOCYTOSIS, leukopenia, thrombocytopenia. **Misc:** Allergic reactions.

Interactions: Concurrent use with drugs that prolong QT interval, including antiarrhythmics, pimozide, erythromycin, clarithromycin, fluoroquinolones, methadone, and tricyclic antidepressants, may ↑ the risk for arrhythmias; concurrent use should be avoided. Additive hypotension with antihypertensives. Additive CNS depression with other CNS depressants, including alcohol, antidepressants, antihistamines, opioids, *sedatives/hypnotics,* and *general anesthetics. Phenobarbital* may ↑ metabolism and ↓ effectiveness of fluphenazine. May ↑ risk of *lithium* toxicity. *Aluminum-containing antacids* may ↓ oral absorption of fluphenazine. May ↓ anti-Parkinson activity of *levodopa* and *bromocriptine.* May ↓ vasopressor response to *epinephrine* and *norepinephrine. Beta-blockers, chlorpromazine, chloroquine, delavirdine, fluoxetine, paroxetine, quinidine, quinine, ritonavir,* and *ropinirole* may ↑ the effects of fluphenazine. ↑ Risk of anticholinergic effects with other *agents having anticholinergic properties,* including *antihistamines, tricyclic antidepressants, disopyramide,* and *quinidine. Metoclopramide* may ↑ risk of extrapyramidal reactions.

Dosage: *Fluphenazine Decanoate:* IM (Adults): 12.5–25 mg initially; may be repeated every 3 wk. Dosage may be slowly ↑ as needed (not to exceed 100 mg/dose).

***Fluphenazine Hydrochloride:* PO (Adults):** 0.5–10 mg/day in divided doses every 6–8 hr (maximum dose = 40 mg/day).

PO (Geriatric Clients or Debilitated Clients): 1–2.5 mg/day initially; ↑ dose every 4–7 days by 1–2.5 mg/day as needed (maximum dose = 20 mg/day).

IM (Adults): 1.25–2.5 mg every 6–8 hr.

Availability (generic available)

Fluphenazine decanoate injection: 25 mg/mL, Canadian: 100 mg/mL. COST: **$$.**
Fluphenazine hydrochloride tablets: 1 mg, 2.5 mg, 5 mg Rx, 10 mg. COST: **$.**
Fluphenazine hydrochloride elixir (orange flavor): 2.5 mg/5 mL. COST: **$.**
Fluphenazine hydrochloride concentrate: 5 mg/mL. **Fluphenazine hydrochloride injection**: 2.5 mg/mL.

- **Geriatric Considerations:** Initial dose reduction; start 1–2.5 mg/day. Sensitivity to adverse effects: sedation and hypotension. ↑ Risk of mortality in elderly with dementia-related psychosis.

- **Pediatric/Adolescent Considerations:** Safety not established <6 mo. Very rarely used in pediatric population.

- **Clinical Assessments:** Monitor BP (lying, standing, sitting), pulse, respiration before and during Rx; ECG. Q and T wave changes possible. Monitor for EPS (akathisia, pseudoparkinsonism, dystonia), tardive dyskinesia, and NEUROLEPTIC MALIGNANT SYNDROME. Periodic CBCs (AGRANULOCYTOSIS), FBS, cholesterol, LFTs, and eye examinations. Monitor weight and BMI before and during Rx. (*See BMI/Metabolic Syndrome, Tools tab.*)

Clinical Tips/Alerts: Long-acting depot (decanoate) may be used after client is stabilized on oral preparation. Decanoate takes longer to reach steady state/stabilization, and it is better to start at lower dose and titrate slowly because of long duration and half-life. Conventional depot antipsychotics have been used in clients who have not reliably taken their medications or home-less who may disappear for periods of time. Risperdal Consta IM (atypical antipsychotic) available for injections every other week (see *Risperidone*).

Flurazepam

(flur-**az**-e-pam) Dalmane, *Apo-Flurazepam, Novoflupam, Somnol*

Classification: *Therapeutic:* Sedatives/hypnotics. *Pharmacological:* Benzodiazepines.

Schedule IV; Pregnancy Category X

Indications: Short-term management of insomnia (<4 wk).

Action: Depresses CNS, probably by potentiating GABA, an inhibitory neurotransmitter.

Pharmacokinetics: *Absorption:* Well absorbed after oral administration. *Distribution:* Widely distributed; crosses blood-brain barrier. Probably crosses placenta and enters breast milk. Accumulation of drug occurs with chronic dosing. *Metabolism and Excretion:* Metabolized by liver; some metabolites have hypnotic activity.

Protein Binding: 97% (active metabolite).

T 1/2: 2.3 hr (half-life of active metabolite may be 30–200 hr).

TIME/ACTION PROFILE (hypnotic activity)

Route	Onset	Peak	Duration
PO	15–45 min	0.5–1 hr	7–8 hr

Contraindicated in: Impaired respiratory function; sleep apnea; hypersensitivity; cross-sensitivity with other benzodiazepines may exist; pre-existing CNS depression; severe uncontrolled pain; angle-closure glaucoma. *Pregnancy:* Infants may experience withdrawal effects. *Lactation:* Enters breast milk; discontinue or bottle-feed.

Use Cautiously in: Hepatic dysfunction (dosage reduction may be necessary); history of suicide attempt or drug dependence; debilitated clients (initial dose reduction may be necessary).

Adverse Reactions/Side Effects: (CAPITALS indicate life-threatening; underlines indicate most frequent.)

CNS: Abnormal thinking, behavior changes, confusion, daytime drowsiness, ↓ concentration, dizziness, hallucinations, headache, lethargy, mental depression, paradoxical excitation, sleep driving. **EENT:** Blurred vision. **GI:** Constipation, diarrhea, nausea, vomiting. **Derm:** Rashes. **Neuro:** Ataxia. **Misc:** Physical dependence, psychological dependence, tolerance.

Interactions: Concurrent use with *alcohol, antidepressants, antihistamines,* and *opioids* may result in additive CNS depression. *Cimetidine, hormonal contraceptives, disulfiram, fluoxetine, isoniazid, ketoconazole, metoprolol, propoxyphene, propranolol,* or *valproic acid* may ↓ metabolism of flurazepam, enhancing its actions. May ↓ efficacy of *levodopa. Rifampin* or *barbiturates* may ↑ metabolism and ↓ effectiveness of flurazepam. Sedative effects may be ↓ by *theophylline*. **Drug-Natural:** Concomitant use of *kava, valerian, chamomile,* or *hops* can ↑ CNS depression.

Dosage: PO (Adults): 15–30 mg at bedtime. **PO (Geriatric Clients or Debilitated Clients):** 15 mg initially, may be ↑.

Availability (generic available)

Capsules: 15 mg, 30 mg. **Tablets:** 15 mg, 30 mg. COST: **$$**

- **Geriatric Considerations:** ↑ Risk of falls; on Beers list. Start with lower dose (15 mg at bedtime). Drug accumulation over time. Better to use shorter-acting hypnotic.
- **Pediatric/Adolescent Considerations:** Safety not established <15 yr.
- **Substance Abuse Considerations:** Drug should be used only for short-term management of insomnia. Psychological/physical dependence possible with prolonged use. With physical dependence, withdrawal symptoms may be severe (convulsions, vomiting, sweating).
- **Clinical Assessments:** Monitor for resolution of insomnia; also for confusion and sedation. Assess client before starting drug for actual addictions or addiction-prone behaviors.

Clinical Tips/Alerts: Long-acting benzodiazepine that accumulates (drug and metabolites) over time and may cause impairment (confusion/drowsiness/memory loss) during the day. Need to taper on discontinuation (weeks to months). Avoid alcohol. Need to be aware of possibility of *complex sleep-related behaviors* (cooking, eating, driving while asleep) and *severe allergic reactions.*

Fluvoxamine

(floo-**voks**-a-meen) Luvox, Luvox CR

Classification: *Therapeutic:* antidepressants, antiobsessive agents; *Pharmacological:* SSRIs; *Pregnancy Category C*

Indications: OCD; Social anxiety disorder (Luvox CR). **Off-Label Use:** Depression, GAD, PTSD.

Action: Inhibits reuptake of serotonin in CNS.

Pharmacokinetics: *Absorption:* 53% absorbed after oral administration. *Distribution:* Excreted in breast milk; enters CNS. Remainder of distribution not known. *Metabolism and Excretion:* Eliminated mostly by kidneys.

T 1/2: 13.6–15.6 hr.

TIME/ACTION PROFILE (improvement on obsessive-compulsive behaviors)

Route	Onset	Peak	Duration
PO	Within 2–3 wk	Several months	Unknown

Contraindicated in: Hypersensitivity to fluvoxamine or other SSRIs; concurrent use or use within 14 days of discontinuing MAOI, alosetron, pimozide, thioridazine, or tizanidine.

Use Cautiously in: Impaired hepatic function; *Pregnancy:* Neonates exposed to SSRI in third trimester may develop drug discontinuation syndrome including respiratory distress, feeding difficulty, and irritability; *Lactation:* Discontinue drug or bottle-feed.

Adverse Reactions/Side Effects: (CAPITALS indicate life-threatening; underlines indicate most frequent.)

CNS: Sedation, dizziness, drowsiness, headache, insomnia, nervousness, weakness, agitation, anxiety, apathy, emotional lability, manic reactions, mental depression, psychotic reactions, syncope. **EENT:** Sinusitis. **Resp:** Cough, dyspnea. **CV:** Edema, hypertension, palpitations, postural hypotension, tachycardia, vasodilation. **GI:** Constipation, diarrhea, dry mouth, dyspepsia, nausea, anorexia, dysphagia, elevated liver enzymes, flatulence, weight gain (unusual), vomiting. **GU:** ↑ Libido/sexual dysfunction. **Derm:** Excessive sweating. **Metab:** Weight gain, loss. **MS:** Hypertonia, myoclonus/twitching. **Neuro:** Hypokinesia/hyperkinesia, tremor. **Misc:** Allergic reactions, chills, flu-like symptoms, tooth disorder/caries, yawning.

Interactions: Serious, potentially fatal reactions (serotonin syndrome) may occur with MAOIs. Smoking may ↑ effectiveness of fluvoxamine. Concurrent use with *tricyclic antidepressants* may ↑ plasma levels of fluvoxamine. ↓ Metabolism and may ↑ effects of some *beta blockers (propranolol)*, *alosetron* (avoid concurrent use), some *benzodiazepines* (avoid concurrent *diazepam*), *carbamazepine, methadone, lithium, theophylline* (↓ dose to 33% of usual dose*), tolbutamide, warfarin,* and *l-tryptophan.* ↑ Blood levels and risk of toxicity from *clozapine* (dosage adjustments may be necessary).

Dosage: PO (Adults): *Initial dose:* 50 mg daily at bedtime; ↑ by 50 mg every 4–7 days until desired effect is achieved. If daily dose >100 mg, give in two equally divided doses or give a larger dose at bedtime (not to exceed 300 mg/day). *Maintenance dose:* Make periodic adjustments to maintain lowest possible dose to control symptoms.

PO (Children 8–17 yr): 25 mg at bedtime, may ↑ by 25 mg/day every 4–7 days (not to exceed 200 mg/day; daily doses >50 mg should be given in divided doses with a larger dose at bedtime). **Hepatic Impairment: PO (Adults):** 25 mg daily at bedtime initially, slower titration and longer dosing intervals should be used.

CR Dosing (Adults) PO: Initial Dose: 100 mg daily at bedtime; ↑ by 50 mg/day every week until symptoms resolve. **Max dose (CR):** 300 mg/day

Availability: Generic; CR-Brand only
Tablets: 25 mg, 50 mg, 100 mg. COST: **$**
CR Tablets: 100 mg, 150 mg. COST: **$$$**

- **Geriatric Considerations:** Lower initial dose and slower titration. ↑ Sensitivity to side effects.
- **Pediatric/Adolescent Considerations:** Safety not established in children <8 yr. Weigh risk against benefit. Monitor for suicidality face-to-face early on and during dosage adjustments.
- **Clinical Assessments:** Monitor for mood improvement and suicidality during treatment.

Clinical Tips/Alerts: Effective in treatment of OCD but may also be helpful with mixed anxiety/depressed states. Sedating qualities helpful with anxiety. Concurrent use with MAOIs or within 2 full weeks of stopping MAOI can be fatal to client (serotonin syndrome). (See *Serotonin Syndrome, Basics tab.*)

Gabapentin

(ga-ba-**pen**-tin) Neurontin

Classification: *Therapeutic:* Analgesic adjuncts, therapeutic, anticonvulsants, mood stabilizers; *Pregnancy Category C*

Indications: Partial seizures (adjunct treatment). Post-herpetic neuralgia. **Off-Label Uses:** Chronic pain. Prevention of migraine headache. Bipolar disorder. Anxiety.

Action: Mechanism of action not known. May affect transport of amino acids across and stabilize neuronal membranes.

Pharmacokinetics: *Absorption:* Well absorbed after oral administration by active transport. At larger doses, transport becomes saturated and absorption ↓ (bioavailability ranges from 60% for a 300-mg dose to 35% for a 1600-mg dose). *Distribution:* Crosses blood-brain barrier; enters breast milk. *Metabolism and Excretion:* Eliminated mostly by renal excretion of unchanged drug.

T 1/2: 5–7 hr (normal renal function); up to 132 hr in anuria.

TIME/ACTION PROFILE (blood levels)

Route	Onset	Peak	Duration
PO	Rapid	2–4 hr	8 hr

Contraindicated in: Hypersensitivity.

Use Cautiously in: Renal insufficiency (↓ dose and/or ↑ dosing interval if CrCl <60 mL/min). **Pregnancy:** Safety not established. **Lactation:** Discontinue drug or bottle-feed.

Adverse Reactions/Side Effects: (CAPITALS indicate life-threatening; underlines indicate most frequent.) **CNS:** Confusion, depression, drowsiness, sedation, anxiety, concentration difficulties (children), dizziness, emotional lability (children), hostility, hyperkinesia (children), malaise, vertigo, weakness. **EENT:** Abnormal vision, nystagmus. **CV:** Hypertension. **GI:** Weight gain, anorexia, flatulence, gingivitis. **MS:** Arthralgia. **Neuro:** Ataxia, altered reflexes, hyperkinesia, paresthesia. **Misc:** Facial edema.

Interactions: *Antacids* may ↓ absorption of gabapentin. ↑ Risk of CNS depression with other *CNS depressants*, including *alcohol, antihistamines, opioids*, and *sedatives/hypnotics. Morphine* ↑ gabapentin levels and may ↑ risk of toxicity; dosage adjustments may be required. **Drug-Natural:** *Kava, valerian, or chamomile* can ↑ CNS depression.

Gabapentin

Dosage: *Epilepsy:* **PO (Adults and Children >12 yr):** 300 mg three times daily initially. Titration may be continued until desired (range 900–1800 mg/day in three divided doses; doses should not be more than 12 hr apart). Doses up to 2400–3600 mg/day have been well tolerated.

PO (Children ≥5–12 yr): 10–15 mg/kg/day in three divided doses initially titrated upward over 3 days to 25–35 mg/kg/day in three divided doses; dosage interval should not exceed 12 hr (doses up to 50 mg/kg/day have been used).

PO (Children 3–4 yr): 10–15 mg/kg/day in three divided doses initially titrated upward over 3 days to 40 mg/kg/day in three divided doses; dosage interval should not exceed 12 hr (doses up to 50 mg/kg/day have been used).

Renal Impairment: PO (Adults and Children >12 yr): *CCr 30–60 mL/min:* 300 mg twice daily; *CCr 15–30 mL/min:* 300 mg once daily; *CCr <15 mL/min:* 300 mg once every other day; further adjustments are based on clinical response.

Availability (generic available)

Capsules: 100 mg, 300 mg, 400 mg. COST: **$–$$**. **Tablets:** 100 mg, 300 mg, 400 mg, 600 mg, 800 mg. COST: **$$–$$$. Oral solution** (cool strawberry anise flavor): 250 mg/5 mL. COST: **$$$**.

- **Geriatric Considerations:** Caution with age-related ↓ renal function.
- **Pediatric/Adolescent Considerations:** Safety not established <3 yr. No known indication or clinical trials for pediatric psychiatric use.
- **Clinical Assessments:** Monitor for improvement in mood, sedation, weight gain. Monitor for suicidality.

[**Clinical Tips/Alerts:** Caution with renal impairment (see creatinine clearance and dosing). Doses need to be divided and intervals should not exceed 12 hr.]

Galantamine

(ga-**lant**-a-meen) Razadyne, Razadyne ER

Classification: *Therapeutic:* Anti-Alzheimer's agents

Pharmacological: Cholinergics (cholinesterase inhibitors); *Pregnancy Category B*

Indications: Mild-to-moderate dementia of Alzheimer's type.

Action: Enhances cholinergic function by reversible inhibition of cholinesterase.

Pharmacokinetics: *Absorption:* Well absorbed (90%) following oral administration.

Distribution: Unknown. *Metabolism and Excretion:* Mostly metabolized by liver; 20% excreted unchanged in urine.
↑ ½: 7 hr.

TIME/ACTION PROFILE (anticholinesterase activity)

Route	Onset	Peak	Duration
PO	Unknown	1 hr	12 hr
PO-ER	Unknown	1 hr	24 hr

Contraindicated in: Hypersensitivity; severe hepatic or renal impairment; *Children and lactation.*

Use Cautiously in: Clients with supraventricular cardiac conduction defects or concurrent use of drugs that may slow heart rate (↑ risk of bradycardia); history of ulcer disease/GI bleeding/concurrent NSAID use; severe asthma or obstructive pulmonary disease; mild to moderate renal impairment (avoid use if CCr <9 mL/min); mild to moderate hepatic impairment (cautious dose titration recommended); may ↑ risk of CV mortality. *Pregnancy:* Use only if potential benefit outweighs potential risk to fetus.

Adverse Reactions/Side Effects: (CAPITALS indicate life-threatening; underlines indicate most frequent.)

CNS: Fatigue, dizziness, headache, syncope. **CV:** Bradycardia, chest pain. **GI:** Anorexia, diarrhea, dyspepsia, flatulence, nausea, vomiting. **GU:** Bladder outflow obstruction, incontinence. **Neuro:** Tremor. **Misc:** Weight loss.

Interactions: Will ↑ neuromuscular blockade from *succinylcholine-type neuromuscular blocking agents.* May ↑ effects of other cholinesterase inhibitors or other cholinergic agonists, including bethanechol. May ↑ effectiveness of anticholinergic medications. Blood levels and effects may be ↑ by ketoconazole, paroxetine, amitriptyline, fluvoxamine, or quinidine.

Dosage: PO (Adults): *Immediate-release tablets:* 4 mg twice daily initially; dose increments of 4 mg should be made at 4-wk intervals up to 12 mg twice daily. Doses up to 16 mg twice daily have been used (range 16–32 mg/day; *extended-release capsules:* 8 mg/day as a single dose in the morning; may be ↑ to 16 mg/day after 4 wk, then up to 24 mg/day after 4 wk; increments based on benefit/tolerability. **Renal Impairment PO (Adults):** *Moderate renal impairment:* Daily dose should not exceed 16 mg.

Hepatic Impairment: PO (Adults): *Moderate hepatic impairment:* Daily dose should not exceed 16 mg.

Availability: Brand only

Immediate-release tablets: 4 mg, 8 mg, 12 mg. COST: **$$. Extended-release capsules**: 8 mg, 16 mg, 24 mg. COST: **$$$. Oral solution**: 4 mg/mL in 100-mL bottles.

- **Geriatric Considerations:** Note dosing for renal impairment.
- **Pediatric/Adolescent Considerations**: Contraindicated.
- **Clinical Assessments:** Assess cognitive functions, MMSE, clock-drawing test periodically. Monitor heart rate for bradycardia.

Clinical Tips/Alerts: See *Dosage for renal* and *hepatic impairment*. Best to titrate slowly because of GI side effects of diarrhea, nausea, and vomiting. Maintain on stable dose for at least 4 weeks before increasing dose. Note: *Dementia clients with psychosis* should not use atypical/conventional antipsychotics because of ↑ risk of mortality.

Psychotropic Drugs H-M

Haloperidol

(ha-loe-**per**-i-dole) Haldol, Haldol Decanoate, Apo-Haloperidol, Haloperidol LA, Novo-Peridol, Peridol, PMS Haloperidol

Classification: *Therapeutic:* Antipsychotics; *Pharmacological:* Butyrophenones;

Pregnancy Category C

Indications: Acute and chronic psychotic disorders including: schizophrenia, manic states, drug-induced psychoses. Schizophrenic clients who require long-term parenteral (IM) antipsychotic therapy. Useful in managing aggressive or agitated clients. Tourette's syndrome. Severe behavioral problems in children which may be accompanied by: unprovoked, combative, explosive hyperexcitability, hyperactivity accompanied by conduct disorders (short-term use when other modalities have failed). Considered second-line treatment after failure with atypical antipsychotic. **Off-Label Use:** Nausea and vomiting from surgery or chemotherapy.

Action: Alters effects of dopamine in CNS. Has anticholinergic and alpha-adrenergic blocking activity. *Therapeutic Effects:* Diminished signs and symptoms of psychoses. Improved behavior in children with Tourette's syndrome or other behavioral problems. **Pharmacokinetics:** *Absorption:* Well absorbed following PO/IM administration. Decanoate salt absorbed slowly and has a long duration of action. *Distribution:* Concentrates in liver. Crosses placenta; enters breast milk. *Metabolism and Excretion:* Mostly metabolized by liver.
Protein Binding: 90%.
T 1/2: 21–24 hr.

TIME/ACTION PROFILE (antipsychotic activity)

Route	Onset	Peak	Duration
PO	2 hr	2–6 hr	8–12 hr
IM	20–30 min	30–45 min	4–8 hr*
IM (decanoate)	3–9 days	Unknown	1 mo

*Effect may persist for several days

Contraindicated in: Hypersensitivity; angle-closure glaucoma; bone marrow depression; CNS depression; severe liver or CV disease (Q-T interval prolonging conditions);

some products contain tartrazine, sesame oil, or benzyl alcohol and should be avoided in clients with known intolerance or hypersensitivity.

Use Cautiously in: Debilitated clients (dose reduction required); cardiac disease; diabetes; respiratory insufficiency; prostatic hyperplasia; CNS tumors; intestinal obstruction; seizures. *Pregnancy:* Safety not established. *Lactation:* Discontinue drug or bottle-feed.

Adverse Reactions/Side Effects: (CAPITALS indicate life-threatening; underlines indicate most frequent.)

CNS: SEIZURES, extrapyramidal reactions, confusion, drowsiness, restlessness, tardive dyskinesia (TD). **EENT:** Blurred vision, dry eyes. **Resp:** Respiratory depression. **CV:** Hypotension, tachycardia. **GI:** Constipation, dry mouth, anorexia, drug-induced hepatitis, ileus, weight gain. **GU:** Urinary retention. **Derm:** Diaphoresis, photosensitivity, rashes. **Endo:** Galactorrhea, amenorrhea. **Hemat:** Anemia, leukopenia. **Metab:** Hyperpyrexia. **Misc:** NEUROLEPTIC MALIGNANT SYNDROME, hypersensitivity reactions.

Interactions: ↑ Hypotension with *antihypertensives, nitrates,* or acute ingestion of *alcohol.* ↑ Anticholinergic effects with *drugs having anticholinergic properties,* including *antihistamines, antidepressants, atropine, phenothiazines, quinidine,* and *disopyramide.* ↑ CNS depression with other *CNS depressants,* including *alcohol, antihistamines, opioid analgesics, and sedative/hypnotics.* Concurrent use with *epinephrine* may result in severe hypotension and tachycardia. May ↓ therapeutic effects of *levodopa.* Acute encephalopathic syndrome may occur when used with *lithium.* Dementia may occur with *methyldopa. Drug-Natural:* Kava, valerian, or chamomile can ↑ CNS depression.

Dosage: **Haloperidol PO (Adults):** 0.5–5 mg two to three times daily. Clients with severe symptoms may require up to 100 mg/day.

PO (Geriatric Clients or Debilitated Clients): 0.5–2 mg twice daily initially; may be gradually increased as needed.

PO (Children 3–12 yr or 15–40 kg): 50 mcg/kg/day in two to three divided doses; may increase by 500 mcg (0.5 mg)/day every 5–7 days as needed (up to 75 mcg/kg/day for nonpsychotic disorders or Tourette's syndrome or 150 mcg/kg/day for psychoses).

IM (Adults): 2–5 mg every 1–8 hr (not to exceed 100 mg/day).

Haloperidol Decanoate: IM (Adults): 10–15 times the previous daily PO dose but not to exceed 100 mg initially, given monthly (not to exceed 300 mg/mo).

HydrOXYzine

(hye-**drox**-i-zeen) Atarax, Hyzine-50, Vistaril, *Multipax, Novohydroxyzin, Apo-Hydroxyzine, Vistaril*

Classification: *Therapeutic:* Antianxiety agents, antihistamines, sedative/hypnotics; *Pregnancy Category C*

Indications: Treatment of anxiety. Preoperative sedation. Antiemetic. Antipruritic. May be combined with opioid analgesics.

Action: Acts as CNS depressant at subcortical level of CNS. Has anticholinergic, antihistaminic, and antiemetic properties. Blocks histamine-1 receptors.

Availability (generic available)

Tablets: 0.5 mg, 1 mg, 2 mg, 5 mg, 10 mg, 20 mg. **Oral concentrate:** 2 mg/mL. COST: **$**. Haloperidol injection: 5 mg/mL. COST: **$**. Haloperidol decanoate injection: 50 mg/mL, 100 mg/mL. COST: **$$**.

● **Geriatric Considerations:** Dosage reduction required; sensitivity to adverse effects (hypotension, sedation). Be aware of interactions (anticholinergic) with other drugs and polypharmacy. Start low and titrate slowly. Often used to treat agitation in dementia. ↑ **Risk of mortality in elderly with dementia-related psychosis.**

● **Pediatric/Adolescent Considerations:** Safety not established; should be second-line Rx. Monitor for sedation, EPS, ataxia. (*See Psychotropic Adverse Effects, Basics tab.*) Off-Label use for agitation, anger, and behavioral dyscontrol as second-line therapy only.

● **Clinical Assessments:** Assess mental status, improvement in positive/negative symptoms; monitor BP/pulse before and during Rx. ECG to rule out CV disease (may cause QT interval changes). Monitor for EPS, NMS, TD. (*See Psychotropic Adverse Effects, Basics tab.*) Whenever weight gain an issue, monitor weight, BMI, FBS, and cholesterol before and during Rx. (*See BMI/Metabolic Syndrome, Tools tab.*)

Clinical Tips/Alerts: Do not use with severe liver or CV disease (QT interval prolongation). Start low and titrate slowly with decanoate because of long duration in the body. Decanoate used often in clients unreliable with taking medications. Note: Risperdal Consta IM (atypical antipsychotic) available (*see Risperidone).*

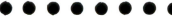

Pharmacokinetics: *Absorption:* Well absorbed following PO/IM administration. *Distribution:* Unknown. Metabolism and *Excretion:* Completely metabolized by liver; eliminated in feces via biliary excretion.

T $\frac{1}{2}$: 3 hr.

TIME/ACTION PROFILE (sedative, antiemetic, antipruritic effects)

Route	Onset	Peak	Duration
PO	15–30 min	2–4 hr	4–6 hr
IM	15–30 min	2–4 hr	4–6 hr

Contraindicated in: Hypersensitivity. *Pregnancy:* Potential for congenital defects (oral clefts and hypoplasia of cerebral hemisphere). *Lactation:* Safety not established.

Use Cautiously in: Severe hepatic dysfunction. *Pregnancy:* Has been used safely *during labor.*

Adverse Reactions/Side Effects: (CAPITALS indicate life-threatening; underlines indicate most frequent.)

CNS: <u>Drowsiness,</u> agitation, ataxia, dizziness, headache, weakness. **Resp:** Wheezing. **GI:** <u>Dry mouth,</u> bitter taste, constipation, nausea. **GU:** Urinary retention. **Derm:** Flushing. **Local:** <u>Pain at IM site,</u> abscesses at IM sites. **Misc:** Chest tightness.

Interactions: Additive CNS depression with other *CNS depressants,* including *alcohol, antidepressants, antihistamines, opioid analgesics, and sedative/hypnotics.* Additive anticholinergic effects with other *drugs possessing anticholinergic properties,* including *antihistamines, antidepressants, atropine, haloperidol, phenothiazines, quinidine,* and *disopyramide.* Can antagonize vasopressor effects of *epinephrine.* ***Drug-Natural:*** Concomitant use of *kava, valerian, or chamomile* can increase CNS depression. Increased anticholinergic effects *with angel's trumpet, Jimson weed, and scopolia.*

Dosage: **PO (Adults):** *Antianxiety:* 25–100 mg four times daily, not to exceed 600 mg/day. *Preoperative sedation:* 50–100 mg single dose. *Antipruritic:* 25 mg three to four times daily.

PO (Children): 2 mg/kg/day divided every 6–8 hr.

IM (Adults): *Preoperative sedation:* 25–100 mg single dose. *Antiemetic, adjunct to opioid analgesics:* 25–100 mg every 4–6 hr as needed. **IM (Children):** 0.5–1 mg/kg/dose every 4–6 hr as needed.

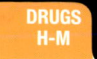
Availability (generic available)
Tablets: 10 mg, 25 mg, 50 mg, 100 mg. COST: **$ Capsules:** Canadian: 10 mg, 25 mg, 50 mg, 100 mg. **Syrup:** 10 mg/5 mL. COST: **$ Oral suspension:** 25 mg/5 mL. COST: **$** Injection: 25 mg/mL, 50 mg/mL.

- **Geriatric Considerations:** Dosage reduction; ↑ sensitivity to adverse effects (delirium, confusion, urinary retention); on Beers list.
- **Pediatric/Adolescent Considerations**: Injection contains benzyl alcohol, which can cause **potentially fatal gasping syndrome in neonates. Monitor for hyperexcitability.**
- **Clinical Assessments:** Assess for anxiety reduction and monitor for excessive sedation.

[**Clinical Tips/Alerts:** Very effective with anxiety-associated pruritic conditions but very sedating. For antianxiety, effective dose may be too sedating. Administer IM hydroxyzine as deep IM.]

Imipramine

(im-**ip**-ra-meen) Tofranil, Tofranil PM, Tipramine, Norfranil, *Apo-Imipramine, Impril, Novopramine*

Classification: *Therapeutic:* Antidepressants; *Pharmacological:* Tricyclic antidepressants; *Pregnancy Category C*

Indications: Various forms of depression. Enuresis in children. **Off-Label Use:** Adjunct in management of chronic pain, incontinence (in adults), vascular headache prophylaxis, cluster headache, insomnia.

Action: Potentiates effect of serotonin and norepinephrine. Has significant anticholinergic properties.

Pharmacokinetics: *Absorption:* Well absorbed from GI tract.

Distribution: Widely distributed. Probably crosses placenta and enters breast milk.

Metabolism and Excretion: Extensively metabolized by liver, mostly on first pass; some conversion to active compounds. Undergoes enterohepatic recirculation and secretion into gastric juices.

Protein Binding: 89%–95%.

T $\frac{1}{2}$: 8–16 hr.

TIME/ACTION PROFILE (antidepressant effect)

Route	Onset	Peak	Duration
PO, IM	Hours	2–6 wk	Weeks

Contraindicated in: Hypersensitivity; cross sensitivity with other antidepressants may occur; angle-closure glaucoma; hypersensitivity to tartrazine or sulfites (in some preparations); recent MI, known history of QTc prolongation, heart failure.
Use Cautiously in: Pre-existing CV disease; seizures or history of seizure disorder; may ↑ risk of suicide attempt/ideation esp. during early treatment or dose adjustment. *Lactation:* Drug present in breast milk; discontinue imipramine or bottle-feed. *Pregnancy:* Studies inconclusive about fetal risk, although there have been reports of congentital malformations; benefits should clearly outweigh risk to justify use of imipramine in pregnancy.
Adverse Reactions/Side Effects: (CAPITALS indicate life-threatening; <u>underlines</u> indicate most frequent.)
CNS: <u>Drowsiness</u>, <u>fatigue</u>, agitation, confusion, hallucinations, insomnia. **EENT:** <u>Blurred vision</u>, <u>dry eyes</u>. **CV:** ARRHYTHMIAS, <u>hypotension</u>, ECG changes. **GI:** <u>Constipation</u>, <u>dry mouth</u>, nausea, paralytic ileus, weight gain. **GU:** Urinary retention, decreased libido. **Derm:** Photosensitivity. **Endo:** Gynecomastia. **Hemat:** Blood dyscrasias.
Interactions: Potentially fatal reactions when used concurrently with *MAOIs;* discontinue MAOI 2 wk before imipramine. Concurrent use *with SSRI antidepressants* should be avoided (*fluoxetine* should be stopped 5 wk before starting imipramine). Concurrent use with *clonidine* may result in hypertensive crisis and should be avoided. Imipramine metabolized in liver by *cytochrome P450 2D6 enzyme* and its action may be affected by drugs that compete for metabolism by this enzyme, including *other antidepressants, phenothiazines, carbamazepine, class 1C antiarrhythmics (propafenone, flecainide);* when used concurrently, dose reduction of one or the other or both may be necessary. Concurrent use of other drugs, including *cimetidine, quinidine, amiodarone, and ritonavir,* that inhibit activity of the enzyme may result in ↑ effects of imipramine. Concurrent use with *levodopa* may result in delayed/↓ absorption of levodopa or hypertension. Blood levels and effects may be ↓ by *rifamycins.* ↑ CNS depression with other CNS *depressants including alcohol, antihistamines, clonidine, opioids, and sedatives/hypnotics. Barbiturates* may alter blood levels and effects. *Adrenergic* and *anticholinergic* side effects may be ↑ with other *agents having these properties. Phenothiazines* or *hormonal contraceptives* ↑ levels and

may cause toxicity. *Cigarette smoking (nicotine)* may increase metabolism and alter effects. **Drug-Natural:** Concomitant use of *kava, valerian,* or *chamomile* can increase CNS depression. ↑ Anticholinergic effects with *Jimson weed* and *scopolia.*

Dosage: PO (Adults): 25–50 mg three or four times daily (not to exceed 300 mg/day); total daily dose may be given at bedtime.

PO (Geriatric Clients): 25 mg at bedtime initially, up to 100 mg/day in divided doses.

PO (Children >12 yr): *Antidepressant:* 25–50 mg/day in divided doses (not to exceed 100 mg/day).

PO (Children 6–12 yr): *Antidepressant:* 10–30 mg/day in two divided doses.

PO (Children ≥6 yr): *Enuresis:* 25 mg once daily 1 hr before bedtime; increase if necessary by 25 mg at weekly intervals to 50 mg in children <12 yr, up to 75 mg in children >12 yr.

IM (Adults): Up to 100 mg/day in divided doses (not to exceed 300 mg/day).

Availability (generic available)
Tablets: 10 mg, 25 mg, 50 mg. Canadian: 75 mg. COST: **$ Capsules:** 75 mg, 100 mg, 125 mg, 150 mg. COST: **$** Injection: 12.5 mg/mL.

● **Geriatric Considerations:** Elderly susceptible to anticholinergic effects; monitor for ↑ sedation, hypotensive effects, urinary retention in males with BPH. Baseline and periodic ECG to monitor for PR/QT prolongation.

● **Pediatric/Adolescent Considerations:** Safety not established in children <6 yr; monitor closely face to face for suicidality early in Rx and during dosage adjustments. Baseline and periodic ECG. Generally considered second-line therapy to SSRI antidepressants.

● **Clinical Assessments:** Evaluate/monitor mood improvement, suicidality. *CV disease:* baseline ECG and repeated ECGs. Overweight: monitor weight, BMI, FBS, cholesterol before and during Rx. (See *BMI/Metabolic Syndrome, Tools tab.*)

[**Clinical Tips/Alerts:** Potentially fatal reaction when used concurrently with MAOI; discontinue MAOI 2 full wk before using imipramine. Fluoxetine should be stopped 5 wk before starting imipramine. (See *Serotonin Syndrome, Basics tab.*) Monitor baseline and periodic ECGs in clients with heart disease.]

Isocarboxazid

(eye-soe-kar-**boks**-a-zid) Marplan

Classification: *Therapeutic:* antidepressants; *Pharmacological:* MAOIs; *Pregnancy Category C*

Indications: Treatment of depression (usually reserved for clients who do not tolerate or respond to other modes of therapy [e.g., tricyclic antidepressants, SSRIs, SNRIs, or electroconvulsive therapy]).

Action: Inhibits enzyme monoamine oxidase, resulting in an accumulation of various neurotransmitters (dopamine, epinephrine, norepinephrine, and serotonin) in the body.

Pharmacokinetics: *Absorption:* Unknown. *Distribution:* Unknown. *Metabolism and Excretion :* Unknown.

T $1/2$: Unknown.

TIME/ACTION PROFILE (antidepressant effect)

Route	Onset	Peak	Duration
PO	Unknown	3–6 wk	Unknown

Contraindicated in: *Lactation.* Hypersensitivity; liver disease; severe renal disease; cerebrovascular disease; CV disease; uncontrolled hypertension; pheochromocytoma; history of severe or frequent headaches; clients undergoing elective surgery requiring general anesthesia (should be discontinued at least 10 days before surgery); excessive consumption of caffeine; concurrent use of meperidine, SSRI antidepressants, SNRI antidepressants, tricyclic antidepressants, tetracyclic antidepressants, nefazodone, trazodone, procarbazine, selegiline, linezolid, carbamazepine, cyclobenzaprine, bupropion, buspirone, sympathomimetics, other MAOIs, dextromethorphan, narcotics, alcohol, general anesthetics, diuretics, tryptophan, or antihistamines; concurrent use of foods containing high concentrations of tyramine; children <16 yr (safety and effectiveness not established).

Use Cautiously in: Clients who may be suicidal or have a history of drug dependency; hyperthyroidism; schizophrenia; bipolar disorder; seizure disorders; diabetes (↑ risk of hypoglycemia). *Pregnancy:* Safety not established.

Adverse Reactions/Side Effects: (CAPITALS indicate life-threatening; <u>underlines</u> indicate most frequent.)

CNS: SEIZURES, <u>dizziness,</u> <u>headache,</u> akathisia, anxiety, ataxia, drowsiness, euphoria, insomnia, restlessness, weakness. **EENT:** <u>Blurred vision.</u> **CV:** HYPERTENSIVE

CRISIS; orthostatic hypotension. **GI:** Nausea, black tongue, constipation, diarrhea, dry mouth. **GU:** Dysuria, sexual dysfunction, urinary incontinence, urinary retention. **Derm:** Photosensitivity.

Interactions: Serious, potentially fatal adverse reactions may occur with concurrent use of other *antidepressants*. Avoid using within 2 wk of each other (wait 5 wk from end of *fluoxetine* therapy). Hypertensive crisis may occur with *amphetamines, methyldopa, levodopa, dopamine, epinephrine, norepinephrine, reserpine, methylphenidate,* or *vasoconstrictors.* Hypertension or hypotension, coma, seizures, respiratory depression, and death may occur with *meperidine* (avoid using within 2–3 wk of MAOI therapy). Concurrent use with *dextromethorphan* may produce psychosis or bizarre behavior. Hypertension may occur with concurrent use of *buspirone;* avoid using within 10 days of each other. Additive hypotension may occur with *antihypertensives, spinal anesthesia, opioids,* or *barbiturates.* Additive hypoglycemia may occur with *insulins* or *oral hypoglycemic agents.* Risk of seizures may be ↑ with *tramadol.* **Drug-Natural:** Serious, potentially fatal adverse effects (serotonin syndrome) may occur with concomitant use of *St. John's wort* and *SAMe.* Hypertensive crises may occur with large amounts of *caffeine*-containing herbs (*cola nut, guarana,* or *maté*). Insomnia, headache, tremor, hypomania may occur with *ginseng.* Hypertensive crises, disorientation, and memory impairment may occur with *tryptophan* or supplements containing *tyrosine* or *phenylalanine.* **Drug-Food:** Hypertensive crisis may occur with ingestion of foods containing high concentrations of *tyramine* (see MAOI Diet, *Tools tab*). Consumption of foods or beverages with high *caffeine* content increases the risk of hypertension and arrhythmias.

Dosage: PO (Adults): 10 mg twice daily; may be increased every 2–4 days by 10 mg, up to 40 mg/day by the end of the first wk, then may increase by up to 20 mg every wk, up to 60 mg/day in two to four divided doses. After optimal response obtained, dose should be slowly decreased to lowest effective amount (40 mg/day or less).

Availability (generic available)
Tablets: 10 mg Rx. COST: $$

● **Geriatric Considerations:** Elderly have greater sensitivity to adverse effects; evaluate for ability to follow diet.
● **Pediatric/Adolescent Considerations:** Approved for use in children ≥16 yr; must follow strict tyramine-restricted diet. Assess early in Rx for suicidality and during dosage adjustments. Generally "last resort" treatment option for adolescent depression.

- **Clinical Assessments:** Assess/monitor for mood improvement, suicidality; monitor BP and pulse before and during Rx; weight and BMI before and during Rx. Other tests: FBS, cholesterol. (*See BMI/Metabolic Syndrome, Tools tab.*)

Clinical Tips/Alerts: Potentially fatal reactions (serotonin syndrome) with concurrent use of other *antidepressants (SSRIs, SNRIs, bupropion, tricyclics, tetracyclics, nefazodone, trazodone), carbamazepine, cyclobenzaprine, sibutramine, procarbazine, or selegiline.* Avoid using within at least 2 wk of each other (wait 5 wk from end of *fluoxetine* therapy). Client **must be willing to follow MAOI (tyramine-restricted) diet** to avoid hypertensive crisis [*emergency*]. (*See MAOI Diet, Tools tab.*) Avoid *meperidine.* Although not a first-line Rx, should be considered for treatment-resistant depression. Associated with weight gain and sedation.

Lamotrigine

(la-**moe**-tri-jeen) Lamictal

Classification: *Therapeutic:* Anticonvulsants, mood stabilizers; *Pregnancy Category C*

Indications: Maintenance treatment of bipolar I disorder. Acute treatment of mood episodes has not been established. Adjunct treatment of partial seizures in adults with epilepsy. Lennox-Gastaut syndrome. Primary generalized tonic-clonic seizures in adults and children ≥2 yr. Conversion to monotherapy in adults with partial seizures receiving single enzyme-inducing antiepileptic drug.

Action: Stabilizes neuronal membranes by inhibiting sodium transport. Inhibits release of glutamate and aspartate.

Pharmacokinetics: *Absorption:* 98% absorbed following oral administration. *Distribution:* Enters breast milk. Highly bound to melanin-containing tissues (eyes, pigmented skin). *Metabolism and Excretion:* Mostly metabolized by liver to inactive metabolites; 10% excreted unchanged by kidneys.

T 1/2: Children taking enzyme–inducing antiepileptic drugs: 7–10 hr; children taking enzyme inducers and valproic acid (VPA): 15–27 hr; children taking VPA: 44–94 hr; adults: 25.4 hr (during chronic therapy of lamotrigine alone).

TIME/ACTION PROFILE (blood levels)

Route	Onset	Peak	Duration
PO	Unknown	1.4–4.8 hr	Unknown

Contraindicated in: Hypersensitivity. *Lactation:* Discontinue drug or stop breast-feeding

Use Cautiously in: Clients with reduced renal function, impaired cardiac function, and impaired hepatic function (lower maintenance doses may be required); prior history of rash to lamotrigine. *Pregnancy:* Exposure during first trimester (may ↑ risk of cleft lip/palate).

Adverse Reactions/Side Effects: (CAPITALS indicate life-threatening; underlines indicate most frequent.)

CNS: Ataxia, dizziness, headache, behavior changes, depression, drowsiness, insomnia, tremor. **EENT:** Blurred vision, double vision, rhinitis. **GI:** Nausea, vomiting. **GU:** Vaginitis. **Derm:** Photosensitivity, rash (higher incidence in children, clients taking VPA, high initial doses, or rapid dose increases), STEVENS-JOHNSON SYNDROME (SJS), TOXIC EPIDERMAL NECROLYSIS. **MS:** Arthralgia. **Misc:** Allergic or hypersensitivity reactions.

Interactions: Concurrent use with *carbamazepine* may result in ↑ levels of lamotrigine and ↑ levels of an active metabolite of *carbamazepine*. Lamotrigine levels are ↓ by concurrent use of *phenobarbital*, *phenytoin*, or *primidone*. Concurrent use with *valproic acid* results in a twofold ↑ in lamotrigine levels, ↑ incidence of rash, and a ↑ in valproic acid level (lamotrigine dose should be ↑ by at least 50%). *Oral contraceptives* may ↑ serum levels of lamotrigine (dose adjustments may be necessary when starting and stopping oral contraceptives).

Dosage: Bipolar disorder & treatment-resistant depression maintenance.

Escalation regimen: **PO (Adults):** *Clients not taking* cabamazepine, valproate, *or other enzyme-inducing drugs:* 25 mg/day for 2 wk, then 50 mg/day for 2 wk, then 100 mg/day for 1 wk, then 200 mg/day. *Clients taking valproate:* 25 mg every other day for 2 wk, then 25 mg/day for 2 wk, then 50 mg/day for 1 wk, then 100 mg/day. *Clients taking* cabamazepine *(or other enzyme inducers)* *but not taking valpo-rate:* 50 mg/day for 2 wk, then 100 mg/day (in divided doses) for 2 wk, then 200 mg/day (in divided doses) for 1 wk, then 300 mg/day (in divided doses) for 1 wk, then up to 400 mg/day (in divided doses).

Dosage adjustment following discontinuation of other psychotropics: **PO (Adults):** *Following discontinuation of other psychotropics:* Maintain previous dose.

Following discontinuation of valproate: 100 mg/day, then increase to 150 mg/day for 1 wk, then 200 mg/day. *Following discontinuation of carbamazepine or other enzyme-inducers:* 400 mg/day for 1 wk, then 300 mg/day for 1 wk, then 200 mg/day. **Availability** (generic available)

Orange 5-wk Titration Starter Kit available by writing NDC number 00173059402 on prescription blank.

Tablets: 25 mg, 100 mg, 150 mg, 200 mg. COST: **$$$$**. **Chewable dispersible tablets:** 2 mg, 5 mg, 25 mg. COST: *Generic* **$$$$**

- **Geriatric Considerations:** Greater sensitivity to adverse effects and may need lower doses.
- **Pediatric/Adolescent Considerations:** Safety and effectiveness in clients <18 yr has not been established. Anecdotal use in pediatrics (> age 8) suggests following same titration schedule as adults, although children's symptoms may remit at lower doses.
- **Clinical Assessments:** Assess mood and monitor for suicidality. Monitor for signs of serious dermatological reaction. *SJS:* Fever, skin rash, blisters or mucous membranes on skin, hives, swollen tongue.

Clinical Tips/Alerts: *Lamotrigine should be discontinued at first sign of rash until medically evaluated for SJS.* Rash usually occurs in first 2 months of Rx; mild rash may be managed with lowering dose. Serious rash, fever, mucosal blisters, or lymphadenopathy requires stopping drug entirely. Inform clients to keep diphenhydramine available for any hint of rash and to take 50 mg en route to hospital emergency department.

Lisdexamfetamine

(lis-dex-am-**fet**-a-meen) Vyvanse

Classification: *Therapeutic:* CNS stimulants; *Schedule II; Pregnancy Category C*

Indications: Prodrug of dextroamphetamine, stimulant for treatment of ADHD in adults and children (ages ≥6 yr).

Action: Blocks reuptake of norepinephrine and dopamine into presynaptic neuron. Pharmacological effects are: CNS and respiratory stimulation, vasoconstriction, mydriasis (pupillary dilation).

Pharmacokinetics: *Absorption:* Well absorbed after oral administration and converted to dextroamphetamine.

Distribution: Widely distributed in body tissues, with high concentrations in the brain and cerebrospinal spinal fluid (CSF). Crosses placenta and enters breast milk. *Metabolism and Excretion:* Some metabolism by liver. Urinary excretion pH-dependent. Alkaline urine promotes reabsorption and prolongs action.

$T_{1/2}$: Children 6–12 yr: 9–11 hr; adults: 10–13 hr (depends on urine pH).

TIME/ACTION PROFILE (CNS stimulation)

Route	Onset	Peak	Duration
PO	1 hr	3.5 hr	8 hr

Contraindicated in: Hyperexcitable states including hyperthyroidism; psychotic personalities; suicidal or homicidal tendencies; glaucoma; chemical dependence; structural cardiac abnormalities (may increase risk of sudden death); during or within 14 days following administration of MAOIs. **Pregnancy:** Potentially embryotoxic.

Use Cautiously in: CV disease (sudden death has occurred in children with structural cardiac abnormalities or other serious heart problems); history of substance abuse (misuse may result in serious CV events/sudden death); hypertension; Tourette's syndrome (may exacerbate tics); seizures.

Adverse Reactions/Side Effects: (CAPITALS indicate life-threatening; underlines indicate most frequent.)

CNS: Hyperactivity, insomnia, irritability, restlessness, tremor, dizziness, headache, tic, somnolence; seizure. **CV:** Palpitations, tachycardia, cardiomyopathy (increased with prolonged use, high doses), hypertension, hypotension. **GI:** Anorexia, constipation, cramps, diarrhea, dry mouth, metallic taste, nausea, vomiting. **GU:** Erectile dysfunction, increased libido. **Derm:** Pyrexia, rash. **Misc:** Psychological dependence.

Interactions: Use with MAOIs or *meperidine* can result in hypertensive crisis. ↑ Adrenergic effects with other adrenergics or thyroid preparations, *Drugs that alkalinize urine (sodium bicarbonate, acetazolamide)* ↑ excretion, ↑ effects, *Drugs that acidify urine (ammonium chloride, large doses of ascorbic acid)* ↓ excretion, ↓ effects, ↑ risk of hypertension and bradycardia with beta blockers, ↑ Risk of arrhythmias with *digoxin. Tricyclic antidepressants* may ↑ effect of amphetamine but may ↑ risk of arrhythmias, hypertension, or hyperpyrexia. **Drug-Natural:** Use with *St. John's wort* may increase serious side effects (avoid concurrent use). **Drug-Food:** *Foods that alkalinize the urine (fruit juices)* can ↑ effect of amphetamine.

Dosage: *ADHD:* **PO (Adults and Children 6–12 yr):** 20 mg/day once daily in the morning; typical dose 30 mg daily in the morning; increase daily dose by 10 mg at weekly intervals up to maximum 70 mg once daily in the morning. Capsules may be opened and contents dissolved in small amount of water if unable to swallow capsule

Availability: Brand only

Capsules: 20 mg, 30 mg, 40 mg, 50 mg, 60 mg, 70 mg. **COST: Brand: $$$**

- **Geriatric Considerations:** No indication for use in geriatric population.
- **Pediatric/Adolescent Considerations:** May have drug-free "holidays" (weekends, summers, school breaks) when using for inattentive type ADHD (summers). Do not use with known cardiac abnormalities.
- **Substance Abuse Considerations:** High potential for abuse; prolonged use may lead to dependence. Dispense sparingly; observe for obtaining for nontherapeutic use or distribution to others.
- **Clinical Assessments:** Monitor BP, pulse, and respiration before and during treatment; monitor for rebound depression/fatigue when medication wears off.

> **Clinical Tips/Alerts:** May cause sudden death with misuse or serious CV adverse events. Do not use with MAOIs (during or within 14 days of MAOI) or meperidine.

Lithium

(**lith**-ee-um) Eskalith, Lithobid, *Carbolith, Duralith, Lithizine*

Classification: *Therapeutic:* Mood stabilizers; *Pregnancy Category D*

Indications: Bipolar disorder: Acute manic episodes, prophylaxis, and maintenance.

Off-Label Use: Schizoaffective disorder, adjunctive treatment of depression.

Action: Alters cation transport in nerve and muscle. May also influence reuptake of neurotransmitters. Inhibits inositol monophosphatase.

Pharmacokinetics: *Absorption:* Completely absorbed after oral administration. *Distribution:* Widely distributed into many tissues and fluids; CSF levels 50% of plasma levels. Crosses placenta; enters breast milk. *Metabolism and Excretion:* Excreted almost entirely unchanged by kidneys.

T $\frac{1}{2}$: 20–27 hr.

TIME/ACTION PROFILE (antimanic effects)

Route	Onset	Peak	Duration
PO, PO-ER	5–7 days	10–21 days	Days

Contraindicated in: Hypersensitivity; severe CV or renal disease; dehydrated or debilitated clients; should be used only where therapy, including blood levels, may be closely monitored; some products contain alcohol or tartrazine and should be avoided in clients with known hypersensitivity or intolerance.

Use Cautiously in: Any amount of cardiac, renal, or thyroid disease; diabetes mellitus. **Pregnancy/Lactation:** Safety not established.

Adverse Reactions/Side Effects: (CAPITALS indicate life-threatening; underlines indicate most frequent.)

CNS: SEIZURES, fatigue, headache, impaired memory, ataxia, sedation, confusion, dizziness, drowsiness, psychomotor retardation, restlessness, stupor. **EENT:** Aphasia, blurred vision, dysarthria, tinnitus. **CV:** ARRHYTHMIAS, ECG changes, edema, hypotension. **GI:** Abdominal pain, anorexia, bloating, diarrhea, nausea, dry mouth, metallic taste. **GU:** Polyuria, glycosuria, nephrogenic diabetes insipidus, renal toxicity. **Derm:** Acneiform eruption, folliculitis, alopecia, diminished sensation, pruritus. **Endo:** Hypothyroidism, goiter, hyperglycemia, hyperthyroidism. **F and E:** Hyponatremia. **Hemat:** Leukocytosis. **Metab:** Weight gain. **MS:** Muscle weakness, hyperirritability, rigidity. **Neuro:** Tremors.

Interactions: May prolong action of *neuromuscular blocking agents.* ↑ Risk of neurological toxicity with *haloperidol* or *molindone. Diuretics, methyldopa, probenecid, fluoxetine,* and *NSAIDs* may ↑ risk of toxicity. Blood levels may be ↑ by *angiotensin-converting enzyme inhibitors.* Lithium may ↑ effects of *chlorpromazine. Chlorpromazine* may mask early signs of lithium toxicity. Hypothyroid effects may be additive with *potassium iodide* or *antithyroid agents. Aminophylline, phenothiazines,* and *drugs containing large amounts of sodium* ↑ renal elimination and ↓ effectiveness. *Psyllium* can ↑ lithium levels. **Drug-Natural:** Caffeine-containing herbs *(cola nut, guarana, mate, tea, coffee)* may ↑ lithium serum levels and efficacy. **Drug-Food:** Large changes in *sodium intake* may alter renal elimination of lithium. ↑ *Sodium intake* will ↑ renal excretion.

Dosage: Precise dosing is based on serum lithium levels. (See *Therapeutic Plasma Levels, Labs tab.*)

PO (Adults and children ≥12 yr): *Tablets/capsules:* 300–600 mg three times daily initially; usual maintenance dose 300 mg three to four times daily. *Slow-release capsules:* 200–300 mg three times daily initially; increased up to 1800 mg/day in divided doses. Usual maintenance dose 300–400 mg three times daily. *Extended-release tablets:* 450–900 mg twice daily *or* 300–600 mg three times daily initially; usual maintenance dose 450 mg twice daily *or* 300 mg three times daily.

PO (Children <12 yr): 15–20 mg (0.4–0.5 mEq)/kg/day in two to three divided doses; dosage may be adjusted weekly.

Availability (generic available)

Capsules: 150 mg, 300 mg, 600 mg. COST: *Generic* **$. Controlled-release tablets:** 300 mg, 450 mg. COST: *Generic* **$. Slow-release tablets:** 300 mg. **Syrup:** 300 mg (8 mEq lithium)/5 mL. COST: **$**

- **Geriatric Considerations:** Initial dose reduction and possibly lower maintence doses due to age-related changes and sensitivity to side effects.
- **Pediatric/Adolescent Considerations:** Not approved <12 yr; use with caution and monitor closely for side effects and suicidality. Children may experience more frequent and severe side effects.
- **Clinical Assessments:** Monitor mental status and mood and for suicidality. Monitor input and output (avoid dehydration). Monitor serum lithium levels twice weekly, then every 3 months once stabilized. Narrow therapeutic window, must monitor for lithium toxicity. Evaluate renal/thyroid function (hypothyroidism), WBC with differential, serum electrolytes, FBS, BMI, cholesterol, weight, before and during Rx. (*See BMI/Metabolic Syndrome, Tools tab.*)

Clinical Tips/Alerts: Multiple side effects can make adherence difficult: tremors, fatigue, impaired memory, polyuria, acne, rash, alopecia. For this reason, although effective, other newer mood stabilizers may be first choice. *Signs of* **lithium toxicity:** (Vomiting, diarrhea, slurred speech, muscle twitching, ↓ coordination); check serum levels immediately (therapeutic levels: acute mania: 1.0–1.5 mEq/L; maintenance: 0.6–1.2 mEq/L). Lithium blood levels should be drawn in the morning about 12 hours after last oral dose and before first morning dose. Weight gain can be significant. *Toxic encephalopathy* possible with concomitant haloperidol. Avoid use with diruetics and NSAIDs.

Lorazepam

(lor-**az**-e-pam) Ativan, *Apo-Lorazepam, Novo-Lorazem, Nu-Loraz*

Classification: *Therapeutic:* Analgesic adjuncts, antianxiety agents, sedative/ hypnotics. *Pharmacological:* Benzodiazepines. *Schedule IV. Pregnancy Category D*

Indications: Anxiety disorder (oral). Preoperative sedation (injection). Decreases pre-operative anxiety and provides amnesia. **Off-Label Use:** IV : Antiemetic before chemotherapy. Insomnia, panic disorder, as an adjunct with acute mania or acute psychosis.

Action: Depresses the CNS, probably by potentiating GABA, an inhibitory neuro-transmitter.

Pharmacokinetics: *Absorption:* Well absorbed following oral administration. Rapidly and completely absorbed following IM administration. Sublingual absorption more rapid than oral and similar to IM. *Distribution:* Widely distributed. Crosses blood-brain barrier. Crosses placenta; enters breast milk. *Metabolism and Excretion:* Highly metabolized by liver.

$T\ 1/2$: Full-term neonates: 18–73 hr; older children: 6–17 hr; Adults: 10–16 hr.

TIME/ACTION PROFILE (sedation)

Route	Onset	Peak	Duration
PO	15–60 min	1–6 hr	8–12 hr
IM	30–60 min	1–2 hr*	8–12 hr
IV	15–30 min	15–20 min	8–12 hr

*Amnestic response

Contraindicated in: Hypersensitivity; cross sensitivity with other benzodiazepines may exist; comatose clients or those with pre-existing CNS depression; uncontrolled severe pain; angle-closure glaucoma; severe hypotension; sleep apnea. **Pregnancy/ Lactation:** Use in pregnancy and lactation may cause CNS depression, flaccidity, feeding difficulties, hypothermia, seizures, and respiratory problems in the neonate.
Lactation: Recommend to discontinue drug or bottle-feed.

Use Cautiously in: *Severe* hepatic/renal/pulmonary impairment; myasthenia gravis; depression; psychosis; history of suicide attempt or drug abuse; COPD; sleep apnea; lower doses recommended for debilitated clients; hypnotic use should be short-term.
OVERDOSE: Administer flumazenil (do not use with clients with seizure disorder).
May induce seizures.

Adverse Reactions/Side Effects: (CAPITALS indicate life-threatening; <u>underlines</u> indicate most frequent.)
CNS: <u>Dizziness,</u> <u>drowsiness,</u> <u>lethargy,</u> hangover, headache, ataxia, slurred speech, forgetfulness, confusion, mental depression, rhythmic myoclonic jerking in pre-term infants, paradoxical excitation. **EENT:** Blurred vision. **Resp:** Respiratory depression. **CV: Rapid IV use only:** APNEA, CARDIAC ARREST, bradycardia, hypotension. **GI:** Constipation, diarrhea, nausea, vomiting, weight gain (unusual). **Derm:** Rashes. **Misc:** Physical dependence, psychological dependence, tolerance.

Interactions: Additive CNS depression with *other CNS depressants,* including *alcohol, antihistamines, antidepressants, opioid analgesics, clozapine,* and other *sedative/ hypnotics* including other benzodiazepines. May ↓ efficacy of *levodopa. Smoking* may ↑ metabolism and ↓ effectiveness. *Valproate* can ↑ serum concentrations and ↓ clearance (↓ dose by 50%). *Probenecid* may ↓ metabolism of lorazepam, enhancing its actions (↓ dose by 50%). *Oral contraceptives* may ↑ clearance and ↓ concentration of lorazepam. ***Drug-Natural:*** Concomitant use of *kava, valerian,* or *chamomile* can ↑ CNS depression.

Dosage: **PO (Adults):** *Anxiety:* 1–3 mg two to three times daily (up to 10 mg/day; typically do not exceed 6 mg/day due to dependence and withdrawal factors). *Insomnia:* 2–4 mg at bedtime.
PO (Geriatric Clients or Debilitated Clients): *Anxiety:* 0.5–2 mg/day in divided doses initially. *Insomnia:* 0.25–1 mg initially, increased as needed.
PO (Children): *Anxiety/sedation:* 0.02–0.1 mg/kg/dose (not to exceed 2 mg) every 4–8 hr. **PO (Infants):** *Anxiety/sedation:* 0.02–0.1 mg/kg/dose (not to exceed 2 mg) every 4–8 hr. **SL (Adults and adolescents > 18 yr):** *Anxiety:* 2–3 mg/day in divided doses, not to exceed 6 mg/day. **SL (Geriatric Clients and Debilitated Clients):** 0.5 mg/day, dose may be adjusted as necessary.
Availability (generic available)
Tablets: 0.5 mg, 1 mg, 2 mg. COST **$$. Concentrated oral solution:** 0.5 mg/5 mL, 2 mg/mL. COST **$$. Sublingual tablets:** Canadian: 0.5 mg, 1 mg, 2 mg. **Injection:** 2 mg/mL, 4 mg/mL. COST: **$$.**

● **Geriatric Considerations:** Lower doses recommended; more sensitive to adverse effects (drowsiness, dizziness); ↑ risk for falls.

- **Pediatric/Adolescent Considerations**: Use cautiously in children under 12 yr. In ↑ doses, benzyl alcohol in injection may cause potentially fatal "gasping syndrome" in neonates.
- **Substance Abuse Considerations**: ↑ Risk for psychological/physical dependence with long-term use.
- **Clinical Assessments**: Evaluate level of anxiety before and during Rx and level of anxiety reduction.

Clinical Tips/Alerts: Useful with agitated client. After high-dose, long-term use, this shorter-acting benzodiazepine will require a slow taper. Requires more frequent dosing than a long-acting benzodiazepine with greater chance of withdrawal symptoms. Best for short-term Rx, using an SSRI for chronic anxiety. May contribute to increased agitation and confusion in the elderly.

Loxapine

(lox-a-peen) Loxitane C, Loxitane IM, *Loxapac*

Classification: *Therapeutic*: Antipsychotics (conventional); *Pregnancy Category C*

Indications: Schizophrenia; considered second-line treatment after failure of atypical antipsychotic. **Off-Label Use**: Other psychotic disorders. Bipolar disorder.

Action: Appears to block dopamine and serotonin at postsynaptic receptor sites in CNS.

Pharmacokinetics: *Absorption*: Well absorbed after IM administration; bioavailability with oral administration approximately 30%. *Distribution*: Unknown. *Metabolism and Excretion*: Extensively metabolized by liver; some conversion to active antipsychotic compounds.

T 1/2: *PO*: 3–4 hr. *IM*: 12 hr.

TIME/ACTION PROFILE (antipsychotic effect)

Route	Onset	Peak	Duration
PO, IM	30 min	1.5–3 hr	12 hr

Contraindicated in: Hypersensitivity or intolerance to loxapine or amoxapine; coma; CNS depression. *Pregnancy*: Safety not established; weigh potential benefit against possible risks to fetus. *Lactation*: Discontinue loxapine or bottle-feed.

Use Cautiously in: Glaucoma; intestinal obstruction; history of seizures; alcoholism; CV disease; impaired liver function; men with prostatic hyperplasia (more prone to urinary retention).

Adverse Reactions/Side Effects: (CAPITALS indicate life-threatening; <u>underlines</u> indicate most frequent.)

CNS: NEUROLEPTIC MALIGNANT SYNDROME, <u>confusion,</u> <u>dizziness,</u> <u>drowsiness,</u> extrapyramidal reactions, headache, insomnia, syncope, TD, weakness. **EENT:** <u>Blurred vision,</u> lens opacities, nasal congestion. **CV:** <u>Orthostatic hypotension,</u> tachycardia. **GI:** Constipation, drug-induced hepatitis, dry mouth, ileus, nausea, vomiting. **GU:** Urinary retention. **Derm:** Dermatitis, edema, facial photosensitivity, pigment changes, rashes, seborrhea. **Endo:** Galactorrhea. **Hemat:** AGRANULOCYTOSIS. **Neuro:** Ataxia. **Misc:** Allergic reactions.

Interactions: Decreases antihypertensive effects of *guanadrel*. Blocks alpha-adrenergic effects of *epinephrine* (may result in hypotension and tachycardia). Additive CNS depression with other *CNS depressants*, including *alcohol, antihistamines, opioid analgesics,* and *sedatives/hypnotics. Antacids* or *adsorbent antidiarrheals* may decrease absorption. Use with *antidepressants* or *MAOIs* may result in prolonged CNS depression and increased anticholinergic effects. ***Drug-Natural:*** Concomitant use of *kava, valerian, skullcap, chamomile,* or *hops* can increase CNS depression.

Dosage: **PO (Adults):** 10 mg twice daily, may be increased gradually over the first 7–10 days as needed and tolerated. Usual maintenance dose 60–100 mg/day. **IM (Adults):** 12.5–50 mg every 4–6 hr as needed and tolerated; some clients respond to twice daily dosing.

Availability (generic available)

Capsules: 5 mg, 10 mg, 25 mg, 50 mg. **Tablets:** COST: **$.** Canadian: 5 mg, 10 mg, 25 mg, 50 mg. **Oral concentrate**: 25 mg/mL. COST: **$ Injection:** 50 mg/mL. Cost: **$**

- **Geriatric Considerations:** Susceptible to adverse effects: moderate to severe sedation, also constipation and urinary retention (males with BPH). Caution with CV disease. ↑ Risk of mortality in elderly with dementia-related psychosis.
- **Pediatric/Adolescent Considerations:** Safety not established <16 yr. No indications.
- **Clinical Assessments:** Monitor mental status, positive and negative symptoms for improvement. Monitor FBS, cholesterol, weight, BMI, before and periodically

Memantine

(me-**man**-teen) Namenda

Classification: *Therapeutic:* Anti-Alzheimer's agents; *Pharmacological:* N-methyl-D-aspartate (NMDA) antagonist; Pregnancy Category B

Indications: Moderate to severe dementia of Alzheimer's type.

Action: Binds to NMDA receptor sites, preventing binding of glutamate, an excitatory neurotransmitter.

Pharmacokinetics: *Absorption:* Well absorbed after oral administration. *Distribution:* Unknown. *Metabolism and Excretion:* 57%–82% excreted unchanged in urine by active tubular secretion moderated by pH-dependent tubular reabsorption. Remainder metabolized; metabolites not pharmacologically active.
$T_{1/2}$: 60–80 hr.

TIME/ACTION PROFILE (blood levels)

Route	Onset	Peak	Duration
PO	Unknown	3–7 hr	12 hr

Contraindicated in: Severe renal impairment.

Use Cautiously in: Moderate renal impairment (consider ↓ dose); concurrent use of other NMDA antagonists (amantadine, rimantadine, ketamine, dextromethorphan); concurrent use of drugs or diets that cause alkaline urine; conditions that ↑ urine pH, including severe urinary tract infections or renal tubular acidosis (lead to ↑ excretion and ↓ levels). **Pregnancy:** Safety not established. **Lactation:** Discontinue drug or bottle-feed.

Adverse Reactions/Side Effects: (CAPITALS indicate life-threatening; underlines indicate most frequent).

CNS: Dizziness, fatigue, headache, sedation. **CV:** Hypertension. **Derm:** Rash. **GI:** Weight gain. **GU:** Urinary frequency. **Hemat:** Anemia.

Interactions: *Medications that* ↑ *urine pH* lead to ↓ excretion and ↑ blood levels *(carbonic anhydrase inhibitors, sodium bicarbonate).*

Dosage: PO (Adults): 5 mg once daily initially, increased at weekly intervals to 10 mg/day (5 mg twice daily), then 15 mg/day (5 mg once daily, 10 mg once daily as separate doses, then to target dose of 20 mg/day [as 10 mg twice daily]).

Availability: Brand only

Tablets: 5 mg, 10 mg, titration package containing 28 5-mg tablets and 21 10-mg tablets. COST: **$$$$**. **Oral solution, sugar-free, alcohol-free (peppermint):** 2 mg/mL in 360–mL bottles.

- **Geriatric Considerations:** Well tolerated in geriatric population.
- **Pediatric/Adolescent Considerations**: Safety not established. No indications.
- **Clinical Assessments:** Assess cognitive function before and during Rx (Mini-Mental State Examination, clock drawing).

[**Clinical Tips/Alerts:** May delay progression but will not improve cognitive function. Family members best source of cognitive stabilization or decline.]

Methylphenidate

(meth-ill-**fen**-i-date) Concerta, Metadate CD, Metadate ER, Methylin, Methylin ER, *PMS-Methylphenidate, Riphenidate*, Ritalin, Ritalin LA, Ritalin-SR, Daytrana Transdermal Patch

Classification: *Therapeutic:* CNS stimulants: *Schedule II; Pregnancy Category C*

Indications: Treatment of ADHD. Symptomatic treatment of narcolepsy. **Off-Label Use:** Management of some forms of refractory depression.

Action: Produces CNS and respiratory stimulation with weak sympathomimetic activity. Enhances dopamine and norepinephrine in dorsolateral prefrontal cortex of brain.

Pharmacokinetics: *Absorption:* Slow and incomplete after oral administration; absorption of sustained or extended-release tablet (SR) delayed and provides continuous release. *Metadate CD, Concerta, Ritalin LA:* Provides initial rapid release followed by a second continuous release (biphasic release). *Distribution:* Unknown. *Metabolism and Excretion:* Mostly metabolized (80%) by liver.

$T \frac{1}{2}$: 2–4 hr.

TIME/ACTION PROFILE (CNS stimulation)

Route	Onset	Peak	Duration
PO	Unknown	1–3 hr	4–6 hr
PO-ER	Unknown	4–7 hr	3–12 hr*
Transdermal	Unknown	4–5 hr	3–9 hr

*Depends on formulation

Contraindicated in: Hypersensitivity; hyperexcitable states; hyperthyroidism; clients with psychotic personalities or suicidal or homicidal tendencies; Tourette's syndrome; glaucoma; motor tics; concurrent use or use within 14 days of MAOIs.

Use Cautiously in: History of CV disease; hypertension; diabetes mellitus; debilitated clients; continual use (may result in psychological or physical dependence); seizure disorders (may lower seizure threshold); Concerta product should be used cautiously in clients with esophageal motility disorders or severe GI narrowing (may increase risk of obstruction); **Pregnancy/Lactation:** Safety not established.

Adverse Reactions/Side Effects: (CAPITALS indicate life-threatening; underlines indicate most frequent.)

CNS: Hyperactivity, insomnia, restlessness, tremor, dizziness, headache, irritability. **EENT:** Blurred vision. **CV:** Hypertension, palpitations, tachycardia, hypotension. **GI:** Anorexia, constipation, cramps, diarrhea, dry mouth, metallic taste, nausea, vomiting. **Derm:** Rashes. **Neuro:** Akathisia, dyskinesia. **Misc:** Fever, hypersensitivity reactions, physical dependence, psychological dependence, suppression of weight gain (children), tolerance.

Interactions: ↑ Sympathomimetic effects with other *adrenergics*, including *vasoconstrictors* and *decongestants*. Use with *MAOIs* or *vasopressors* may result in hypertensive crisis (concurrent use or use within 14 days of MAOIs is contraindicated). Metabolism of *warfarin*, *phenytoin*, *phenobarbital*, *primidone*, *SSRIs*, and *tricyclic antidepressants* may be ↓ and effects ↑. Avoid concurrent use with *pimozide* (may mask cause of tics). Concurrent use with *clonidine* may result in serious ECG abnormalities (40% dose reduction of methylphenidate necessary). **Drug-Natural:** Use with caffeine-containing herbs *(guarana, tea, coffee)* ↑ stimulant effect. *St. John's wort* may increase serious side effects (concurrent use not recommended). **Drug-Food:** Excessive use of caffeine-containing foods or beverages *(coffee, cola, tea)* may cause ↑ CNS stimulation.

Dosage: PO (Adults): *ADHD*: 5–20 mg two to three times daily as prompt-release tablets. When maintenance dose determined, may change to extended-release formulation. *Narcolepsy:* 10 mg two to three times daily; maximum dose 60 mg/day. **PO (Children >6 yr):** *Prompt-release tablets*: 0.3 mg/kg/dose or 2.5–5 mg before breakfast and lunch; increase by 0.1 mg/kg/dose or by 5–10 mg/day at weekly intervals (not to exceed 60 mg/day or 2 mg/kg/day). When maintenance dose determined, may change to extended-release formulation. *Ritalin SR, Metadate ER:* May be used in place of prompt-release tablets when the 8-hour dosage corresponds to the titrated 8-hour dosage of the prompt-release tablets. *Ritalin LA:* Can be given once daily in place of twice-daily regimen at same total dose or in place of SR product at same dose. *Concerta (clients who have not taken methylphenidate previously):* 18 mg once daily in the morning initially, may be titrated as needed up to 54 mg/day. *Concerta (clients currently taking other forms of methylphenidate):* 18 mg once daily in the morning if previous dose was 5 mg two to three times daily or 20 mg daily as SR product; 36 mg once daily in the morning if previous dose was 10 mg two to three times daily or 40 mg daily as SR product; 54 mg once daily in the morning if previous dose was 15 mg two to three times daily or 60 mg once daily as SR product. *Metadate CD:* 20 mg once daily. Dosage may be adjusted in weekly 20-mg increments to a maximum of 60 mg/day taken once daily in the morning. *Daytrana Transdermal Patch:* 10-mg patch daily 2 hours before desired effect; may increase to next-size patch every week. Max: 30-mg patch per day.

Availability (generic available)

Immediate-release tablets: 5 mg, 10 mg, 20 mg. COST: *Generic* **$ to $$**. **Extended-release tablets (Metadate ER, Methylin ER):** 10 mg, 20 mg. **Extended-release tablets (Concerta):** 18 mg, 27 mg, 36 mg, 54 mg. COST: **$$$$**. **Sustained-release tablets (Ritalin SR):** 20 mg. COST: **$$$**. **Extended-release capsules (Metadate CD):** 10 mg, 20 mg, 30 mg. COST: **$$$$**. **Extended-release capsules (Ritalin LA):** 10 mg, 20 mg, 30 mg, 40 mg. COST: **$$$$**. **Chewable tablets (Methylin) (grape flavor):** 2.5 mg, 5 mg, 10 mg. COST: **$**. **Oral solution (Methylin) (grape flavor):** 5 mg/5 mL, 10 mg/5 mL. COST: **$$**. **Daytrana Transdermal Patch:** 10 mg, 15 mg, 20 mg, 30 mg. COST: **$–$$$**.

- **Geriatric Considerations:** Use with caution; also history of hypertension or CV diease.
- **Pediatric/Adolescent Considerations:** Monitor for mood lability, hyperexcitability, and rebound hyperactivity. Adolescents have been known to "share" and sell these medications; monitor closely.

**DRUGS
H–M**

- **Substance Abuse Considerations:** Psychological/physical dependence possible with long-term use. High dependence and abuse potential.
- **Clinical Assessments:** Monitor BP, pulse, respirations before and during Rx; also CBC with differential and platelets periodically. Monitor height and weight in children.
- **Clinical Tips/Alerts:** Concurrent use with an MAOI may result in hypertensive crisis; do not use within 14 days of an MAOI. May experience euphoria and then rebound depression as medication wears off; will need frequent rest periods. Do not use in psychotic clients or those with suicidal/homicidal tendencies or Tourette's syndrome. *Daytrana patch:* Remove approximately 9 hr after applied; observe for contact sensitization (redness, papules, etc.); and discontinue if sensitization develops; fully read prescribing information to ensure propr application and use.

Mirtazapine

(meer-**taz**-a-peen) Remeron, Remeron Soltabs

Classification: *Therapeutic:* antidepressants. *Pharmacological:* tetracyclic antidepressants. **Pregnancy Category C**

Indications: Major depressive disorder. **Off-Label Use:** Panic disorder. GAD. posttraumatic stress disorder.

Action: Blocks various serotonin receptors, blocks histamine receptors, boosts serotonin and norepinephrine/noradrenaline independent of norepinephrine and serotonin reuptake blockade.

Pharmacokinetics: *Absorption:* Well absorbed but rapidly metabolized, resulting in 50% bioavailability. *Distribution:* Unknown. *Metabolism and Excretion:* Extensively metabolized by liver (P450 2D6, 1A2, and 3A enzymes involved); metabolites excreted in urine (75%) and feces (15%).
Protein Binding: 85%.
T $1/2$: 20–40 hr.

TIME/ACTION PROFILE (antidepressant effect)

Route	Onset	Peak	Duration
PO	1–2 wk	6 wk or more	Unknown

Contraindicated in: Hypersensitivity; concurrent MAOI therapy.

Use Cautiously in: History of seizures; history of suicide attempt; may ↑ risk of suicide attempt/ideation esp. during early treatment or dose adjustment; history of mania/hypomania; clients with hepatic or renal impairment. *Pregnancy:* Safety not established. *Lactation:* Discontinue drug or bottle-feed.

Adverse Reactions/Side Effects: (CAPITALS indicate life-threatening; underlines indicate most frequent.)

CNS: Drowsiness, abnormal dreams, abnormal thinking, agitation, anxiety, apathy, confusion, dizziness, malaise, weakness. **EENT:** Sinusitis. **Resp:** Dyspnea, increased cough. **CV:** Edema, hypotension, vasodilation. **GI:** Constipation, dry mouth, increased appetite, abdominal pain, anorexia, elevated liver enzymes, nausea, vomiting. **GU:** Urinary frequency. **Derm:** Pruritus, rash. **F and E**: Increased thirst. **Hemat:** AGRANULOCYTOSIS. **Metab:** Weight gain, hypercholesterolemia, increased triglycerides. **MS:** Arthralgia, back pain, myalgia. **Neuro:** Hyperkinesia, hypesthesia, twitching. **Misc:** Flu-like syndrome.

Interactions: *May cause hypertension, seizures, and death when used with MAOIs; do not use within 14 days of MAOI therapy.* ↑ CNS depression with other *CNS depressants,* including *alcohol* and *benzodiazepines.* Drugs affecting *P450 enzymes, CYP2D6, CYP1A2,* and *CYP3A4* may alter the effects of mirtazapine. *Drug-Natural:* Concomitant use of *kava, valerian, skullcap, chamomile,* or *hops* can ↑ CNS depression. ↑ Risk of serotonergic side effects including serotonin syndrome with *St. John's wort* and *SAMe.*

Dosage: PO (Adults): 15 mg/day as a single bedtime dose initially; may be increased every 1–2 wk up to 45 mg/day.

Availability (generic available)

Tablets: 15 mg, 30 mg, 45 mg. COST: *Generic* **$**. **Orally disintegrating tablets (orange flavor):** 15 mg, 30 mg, 45 mg. COST: *Generic* **$$**.

- **Geriatric Considerations:** ↑ Sensitivity to CNS effects and oversedation. Begin at lower doses and titrate carefully.
- **Pediatric/Adolescent Considerations:** Safety not established. Suicide risk may be greater in chilren or adolescents; assess and monitor closely for suicidality. Has been used off label to improve sleep and appetite in children with ADHD. Monitor closely for changes in mood and agitation.
- **Clinical Assessments:** Assess and monitor CBC and LFTs before and during treatment. Assess mental status for mood improvement; assess for suicidal ideations

esp. early and during dosage adjustments. Monitor weight, BMI, FBS, and choles-terol before and during treatment. *(See BMI/Metabolic Syndrome, Tools tab.)*

[**Clinical Tips/Alerts:** Do not use within 14 days of an MAOI, potentially fatal reaction. There may be significant weight gain and sedation. Has less tendency to cause sexual dysfunction. Helpful with anxious client and insominia.]

Molindone

(**moe**-lin-done) Moban

Classification: *Therapeutic:* Antipsychotics (conventional); *Pregnancy Category unknown*

Indications: Schizophrenia; second-line treatment, after failure with atypical antipsychotics. **Off-Label Use:** Other psychotic disorders. Bipolar disorder.

Action: Blocks effects of dopamine in reticular-activating and limbic systems of brain.

Pharmacokinetics: *Absorption:* Rapidly absorbed following oral administration. *Distribution:* Appears to be widely distributed; probably enters CNS and enters breast milk.

Metabolism and Excretion: Mainly (>90%) metabolized by liver. Small amounts (<3%) excreted unchanged by kidneys.

T $^1/_2$: 1.5 hr.

TIME/ACTION PROFILE (peak = blood levels; duration = antipsychotic effects)

Route	Onset	Peak	Duration
PO	Unknown	1.5 hr	24–36 hr

Contraindicated in: Hypersensitivity to molindone; cross sensitivity with other antipsychotics may exist; severe nervous system depression. *Lactation:* Discontinue drug or bottle-feed.

Use Cautiously in: Diabetes mellitus; respiratory disease; prostatic hyperplasia; CNS tumors; epilepsy; intestinal obstruction; *Pregnancy:* Safety not established.

Adverse Reactions/Side Effects: (CAPITALS indicate life-threatening; underlines indicate most frequent.)

CNS: NEUROLEPTIC MALIGNANT SYNDROME, extrapyramidal reactions, sedation, depression, dizziness, euphoria, headache, insomnia, TD. **EENT:** Blurred vision, dry

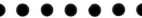

eyes, nasal congestion. **CV:** Hypotension, tachycardia. **GI:** <u>Constipation, dry mouth,</u> anorexia, drug-induced hepatitis, nausea. **Derm:** Photosensitivity, rashes. **Endo:** Galactorrhea, increased libido, irregular menses. **Misc:** Allergic reactions.

Interactions: Additive CNS depression with other *CNS depressants*, including *alcohol, antihistamines, antidepressants, MAOIs, opioid analgesics*, and *sedative/hypnotics*. Additive anticholinergic properties with *agents having anticholinergic effects*, including *phenothiazines, haloperidol, antihistamines, MAOIs*, and *disopyramide*. Encephalopathy may occur with *lithium. Molindone* may mask early signs of lithium toxicity. May negate beneficial effects of *levodopa.* ***Drug-Natural:*** Concomitant use of *kava, valerian, skullcap, chamomile,* or *hops* can increase CNS depression.

Dosage: PO (Adults): 50–75 mg/day in three to four divided doses initially; may be increased to 100 mg/day after 3–4 days. *Usual maintenance dose* 5–25 mg three to four times daily. (Divided doses up to 225 mg/day have been used in severe psychoses.)

PO (Adults: Elderly or Debilitated): Initiate therapy at lower doses.

Availability: Brand only

Tablets: 5 mg, 10 mg, 25 mg, 50 mg, 100 mg. COST: **$$$**

- **Geriatric Considerations:** Lower initial doses recommended. ↑ Risk of mortality in elderly with dementia-related psychosis.
- **Pediatric/Adolescent Considerations**: Safety not established. No indications for use.
- **Clinical Assessments:** Assess mental status before and during Rx; also positive and negative symptoms. Monitor weight, BMI, FBS, cholesterol, LFTs, eye examinations before and during Rx. (*See BMI/Metabolic Syndrome, Tools tab.*) Monitor for EPS, NMS, TD during Rx. (See *Psychotropic Adverse Effects, Basics tab.*) Monitor white blood cells (WBCs) periodically during Rx (WBCs <4000: discontinue medication, consider other Rx or use again when WBCs >4000).

Clinical Tips/Alerts: Molindone less likely to cause weight gain than other conventionals, but EPS may be a problem. Serum prolactin may be elevated (galactorrhea, irregular menses).

Psychotropic Drugs N-Q

Nortriptyline

(nor-**trip**-ti-leen) Aventyl, Pamelor

Classification: *Therapeutic:* Antidepressants; *Pharmacological:* Tricyclic antidepressants; *Pregnancy Category D*

Indications: Major depressive disorder. **Off-Label Use:** Management of chronic neurogenic pain, anxiety, insomnia.

Action: Potentiates effect of norepinephrine/noradrenaline. Has significant anticholinergic properties.

Pharmacokinetics: *Absorption:* Well absorbed after oral administration. *Distribution:* Widely distributed. Enters breast milk in small amounts; probably crosses placenta. *Metabolism and Excretion:* Extensively metabolized by liver, much of it on its first pass. Some is converted to active compounds. Undergoes enterohepatic recirculation and secretion into gastric juices.

Protein Binding: 92%.

T 1/2: 18–28 hr.

TIME/ACTION PROFILE (antidepressant effect)

Route	Onset	Peak	Duration
PO	2–3 wk	6 wk	Unknown

Contraindicated in: Hypersensitivity; angle-closure glaucoma; alcohol intolerance (solution only).

Use Cautiously in: Pre-existing CV disease; history of seizures; asthma; may ↑ risk of suicide attempt/ideation, esp. during early treatment or dose adjustment; risk may be greater in children and adolescents. *Pregnancy:* Use only if clearly needed and maternal benefits outweigh risk to fetus. *Lactation:* May result in sedation in infant; discontinue drug or bottle-feed. Pre-existing CV disease. Geriatric men with prostatic hyperplasia may be more susceptible to urinary retention.

Adverse Reactions/Side Effects: (CAPITALS indicate life-threatening; underlines indicate most frequent):

CNS: Drowsiness, fatigue, lethargy, agitation, confusion, extrapyramidal reactions, hallucinations, headache, insomnia. **EENT:** Blurred vision, dry eyes, dry mouth. **CV:** ARRHYTHMIAS, hypotension, ECG changes. **GI:** Constipation, nausea, paralytic

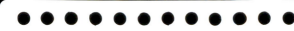

ileus, unpleasant taste, weight gain. **GU:** Urinary retention. **Derm:** Photosensitivity. **Endo:** Gynecomastia. **Hemat:** Blood dyscrasias.

Interactions: May cause fatal reaction when used with *MAOIs* (avoid concurrent use: discontinue 2 wk before starting nortriptyline). May prevent therapeutic response to most *antihypertensives*. Hypertensive crisis may occur with *clonidine*. ↑ CNS depression with other *CNS depressants*, including *alcohol, antihistamines, opioids,* and *sedative/hypnotics.* Adrenergic effects may be ↑ with other *adrenergic agents,* including *vasoconstrictors* and *decongestants.* ↑ Anticholinergic effects with other *drugs possessing anticholinergic properties,* including *antihistamines, antidepressants, atropine, haloperidol, phenothiazines, quinidine,* and *disopyramide. Cimetidine, fluoxetine,* or *hormonal contraceptives* ↑ blood levels and risk of toxicity. ↑ Risk of agranulocytosis with *antithyroid agents.* **Drug-Natural:** Concomitant use of *kava, valerian,* or *chamomile* can ↑ CNS depression. *St. John's wort* may ↓ serum concentrations and efficacy. ↑ Anticholinergic effects with *Jimson weed* and *scopolia.*

Dosage: PO (Adults): 25 mg three to four times daily, up to 150 mg/day.

PO (Geriatric Clients): 30–50 mg/day in divided doses or as a single dose.

Availability (generic available)

Capsules: 10 mg, 25 mg, 50 mg, 75 mg. COST: **$. Oral Solution:** 10 mg/5 mL. COST: **$$.**

- **Geriatric Considerations:** Initial dose reduction; sensitive to adverse effects, esp. cholinergic, CV; risk of falls due to drowsiness/sedation, hypotension. Monitor for confusional states. Existing BPH ↑ urinary retention.
- **Pediatric/Adolescent Considerations:** Safety and efficacy not established; must evaluate benefits versus risk. ↑ Risk of suicidality in children, adolescents, young adults. Not approved for use in pediatrics.
- **Clinical Assessments:** Monitor for mental status, change in mood, and suicidality early on and during dosage adjustments. Monitor BP and pulse and baseline ECG and periodically with CV disease or geriatric client. Monitor weight, BMI, FBS, cholesterol (see *BMI/Metabolic Syndrome, Tools tab).* Serum levels may be monitored: Therapeutic plasma concentration range is 50–150 ng/mL.

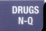

DRUGS N–Q

Olanzapine

(oh-**lan**-za-peen) Zyprexa, Zydis, Symbyax *(combination with fluoxetine)*

Classification: Therapeutic: Antipsychotics (atypical), mood stabilizers; Pharmacological: Thienobenzodiazepines; *Pregnancy Category C*

Indications: Long-term treatment/maintenance of schizophrenia. Bipolar I, acute manic or mixed episodes (monotherapy) (may be used with lithium or valproate); long-term maintenance therapy of bipolar disorder, agitation due to schizophrenia or bipolar I mania **(IM)**. **Symbyax:** Depressive episodes associated with bipolar disorder. **Off-Label Use:** Management of anorexia nervosa. Treatment of nausea and vomiting related to highly emetogenic chemotherapy.

Action: Antagonizes dopamine and serotonin type 2 in the CNS. Also has anticholinergic, antihistaminic, and anti-alpha$_1$ adrenergic effects.

Pharmacokinetics: *Absorption:* Well absorbed but rapidly metabolized by first-pass effect, resulting in 60% bioavailability. Conventional tablets and orally disintegrating tablets (Zydis) are bioequivalent. IM administration results in significantly higher blood levels (five times that of oral).

Distribution: Extensively distributed. *Metabolism and Excretion:* Highly metabolized (mostly by the hepatic P450 CYP 1A2 system); 7% excreted unchanged in urine.

Protein Binding: 93%.

T $1/2$: 21–54 hr.

TIME/ACTION PROFILE (antipsychotic effects)

Route	Onset	Peak*	Duration
PO	Unknown	6 hr	Unknown
IM	Rapid	15–45 min	2–4 hr

* blood levels

Contraindicated in: Hypersensitivity. **Lactation:** Discontinue drug or bottle-feed. Orally disintegrating tablets only: Phenylketonuria (orally disintegrating tablets contain aspartame).

Clinical Tips/Alerts: Tricyclic antidepressants not considered first-line treatment but helpful with chronic pain. Do not use concurrently with MAOI or within 14 days; may cause serotonin syndrome and fatal reaction. (See *Serotonin Syndrome, Basics tab.*)

Use Cautiously in: Clients with hepatic impairment; clients at risk for aspiration; CV or cerebrovascular disease; history of seizures; history of attempted suicide; diabetes or risk factors for diabetes (may worsen glucose control); prostatic hyperplasia; angle-closure glaucoma; history of paralytic ileus; dysphagia and aspiration have been associated with antipsychotic drug use; use with caution in clients at risk for aspiration. *Pregnancy:* Safety not established.

Adverse Reactions/Side Effects: (CAPITALS indicate life-threatening; underlines indicate most frequent.)

CNS: NEUROLEPTIC MALIGNANT SYNDROME, SEIZURES, agitation, dizziness, headache, restlessness, sedation, weakness, dystonia, insomnia, mood changes, personality disorder, speech impairment, tardive dyskinesia. **EENT:** Amblyopia, rhinitis, ↑ salivation, pharyngitis. **Resp:** Cough, dyspnea. **CV:** Orthostatic hypotension (↑ with IM), tachycardia, chest pain. **GI:** Constipation, dry mouth, abdominal pain, ↑ appetite, weight loss or gain, nausea, ↑ thirst. **GU:** ↓ Libido, urinary incontinence. **Derm:** Photosensitivity. **Endo:** Hyperglycemia, goiter. **Metab:** Dyslipidema. **MS:** Hypertonia, joint pain. **Neuro:** Tremor. **Misc:** Fever, flu-like syndrome.

Interactions: Effects may be ↓ by concurrent *carbamazepine, omeprazole,* or *rifampin.* ↑ Hypotension may occur with *antihypertensives.* ↑ CNS depression may occur with concurrent use of *alcohol or* other *CNS depressants.* May antagonize effects of *levodopa* or other *dopamine agonists. Nicotine* can ↓ olanzapine levels.

Dosage: PO (Adults: Most Clients): *Schizophrenia:* 5–10 mg/day initially; may ↑ at weekly intervals by 5 mg/day (not to exceed 20 mg/day). *Bipolar mania:* 10–15 mg/day initially; may ↑ every 24 hr by 5 mg/day (not to exceed 20 mg/day). **PO (Adults: Debilitated or Nonsmoking Female Clients ≥65 yr):** Initiate therapy at 5 mg/day. **IM (Adults):** *Acute agitation:* 5–10 mg, may repeat in 2 hr, then 4 hr later.

Symbyax: *Dosing options:* 6/25, 6/50, 12/25, 12/50 mg/d. Start 6/25 (6 mg olanzapine/25 mg fluoxetine) once daily PO in the evening.

Availability: Brand only

Tablets: 2.5 mg, 5 mg, 7.5 mg, 10 mg, 15 mg, 20 mg. COST: **$$$$.** Orally disintegrating tablets (Zydis): 5 mg, 10 mg, 15 mg, 20 mg. COST: **$$$$.** Powder for injection: 10 mg/vial. COST: **$$$$.** *In combination with:* Fluoxetine (Symbyax). COST: **$$$$.**

✿ **Geriatric Considerations:** Reduce dosage; very sedating (falls). Cerebrovascular adverse events, including stroke, reported in elderly who have dementia-related psychosis, *with* ↑ *risk for mortality.* Not approved for clients with dementia-related psychosis.

● **Pediatric/Adolescent Considerations:** Safety not established. Tablets and Zydis formulations have shown efficacy in clinical trials with children and adolescents with behavioral disturbances.

● **Clinical Assessments:** Monitor weight, BMI, FBS, Hb A₁C, cholesterol before and during treatment. (See *BMI/Metabolic Syndrome, Tools tab.*) CBC, LFTs, and eye examinations periodically. Monitor for EPS, tardive dyskinesia (TD) (rare), and NMS. (See *Psychotropic Adverse Effects, Basics tab.*) Evaluate mental status, mood, and behavior.

Clinical Tips/Alerts: Known for sedation and for ↑ in weight and possibility of diabetes and metabolic syndrome (↑ abdominal fat, hyperglycemia, ↑ lipids). (See *BMI/Metabolic Syndrome, Tools tab.*) Symbyax a combination of olanzapine and fluoxetine *(see also adverse/side effects of fluoxetine).* Zydis orally disintegrating and can be taken with or without water. Monitor for suicidality.

Oxazepam

(ox-**az**-e-pam) Serax, Apo-Oxazepam, Novoxapam

Classification: *Therapeutic:* Antianxiety agents, sedative/hypnotics; *Pharmacological:* Benzodiazepines; *Schedule IV; Pregnancy Category D*

Indications: Management of anxiety, anxiety associated with depression. Symptomatic treatment of alcohol withdrawal.

Action: Depresses the CNS, probably by potentiating GABA, an inhibitory neurotransmitter.

Pharmacokinetics: *Absorption:* Well absorbed following oral administration. *Distribution:* Widely distributed. Absorption slower than with other benzodiazepines. Crosses blood-brain barrier. May cross placenta and enter breast milk. Recommend to discontinue drug or bottle-feed. *Metabolism and Excretion:* Metabolized by liver to inactive compounds. **Protein Binding:** 97%.

T $\frac{1}{2}$: 5–15 hr.

TIME/ACTION PROFILE (sedation)

Route	Onset	Peak	Duration
PO	45–90 min	Unknown	6–12 hr

Contraindicated in: *Pregnancy and lactation*. Hypersensitivity; cross-sensitivity with other benzodiazepines may exist; comatose clients or those with pre-existing CNS depression; uncontrolled severe pain; angle-closure glaucoma; some products contain tartrazine and should be avoided in clients with known intolerance.

Use Cautiously in: Hepatic dysfunction (may be preferred over some benzodiazepines due to short half-life); history of suicide attempts or drug abuse; debilitated clients (initial dosage reduction recommended); severe COPD; myasthenia gravis.

Adverse Reactions/Side Effects: (CAPITALS indicate life-threatening; underlines indicate most frequent.)

CNS: <u>Dizziness</u>, <u>drowsiness</u>, confusion, hangover, headache, impaired memory, mental depression, paradoxical excitation, slurred speech. **EENT:** Blurred vision. **Resp:** Respiratory depression. **CV:** Tachycardia. **GI:** Constipation, diarrhea, drug-induced hepatitis, nausea, vomiting, weight gain (unusual). **GU:** Urinary problems. **Derm:** Rashes. **Hemat:** Leukopenia. **Misc:** Physical dependence, psychological dependence, tolerance.

Interactions: Additive CNS depression with other *CNS depressants*, including *alcohol, antihistamines, antidepressants, opioid analgesics*, and other *sedatives/hypnotics* (including other *benzodiazepines*). May ↓ therapeutic effectiveness of *levodopa*. *Hormonal contraceptives* or *phenytoin* may ↓ effectiveness. *Theophylline* may ↓ sedative effects of oxazepam. ***Drug-Natural:*** Concomitant use of *kava, valerian, skullcap, chamomile,* or *hops* can ↑ CNS depression.

Dosage: PO (Adults): *Antianxiety agent:* 10–30 mg three to four times daily. *Sedative/hypnotic/management of alcohol withdrawal:* 15–30 mg three to four times daily.

PO (Geriatric Clients): 5 mg one to two times daily initially or 10 mg three times daily; may be ↑ as needed.

Availability (generic available)

Capsules: 10 mg, 15 mg, 30 mg COST: **$. Tablets:** Canadian: 10 mg, 15 mg, Canadian: 30 mg.

- **Geriatric Considerations:** On Beers list; ↑ risk for falls and confusion. Start initially with lower dose.
- **Pediatric/Adolescent Considerations:** Dosage not established for 6–12 years; safety not established <6 yr.
- **Substance Abuse Considerations:** Psychological/physical dependence possible with prolonged use/higher dose. This short-acting, low-potency drug is less reinforcing chemically and has less street value than alprazolam or lorazepam.

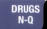

DRUGS N–Q

- **Clinical Assessments:** Assess for continued prescription and physical/psychological dependence.

Clinical Tips/Alerts: Taper drug (0.5 mg every 3–5 days) to avoid withdrawal. Prolonged use requires longer taper. *Withdrawal symptoms include* insomnia, irritability, agitation, headache, tremors. Should be used for acute anxiety; other drugs (SSRIs, e.g., Paxil) should be considered for chronic anxiety (GAD)].

Paliperidone
(pa-li-**per**-i-done) Invega

Classification: *Therapeutic:* Antipsychotics; *Pharmacological:* Benzisoxazoles;

Pregnancy Category C

Indications: Schizophrenia.

Action: May act by antagonizing dopamine and serotonin in the CNS. Paliperidone is active metabolite of risperidone.

Pharmacokinetics: *Absorption:* 28% absorbed following oral administration; food ↑ absorption. *Distribution:* Unknown. *Metabolism and Excretion:* 59% excreted unchanged in urine; 32% excreted in urine as metabolites.

$T^{1/2}$: 23 hr.

TIME/ACTION PROFILE (blood levels)

Route	Onset	Peak	Duration
PO	Unknown	24 hr	24 hr

Contraindicated in: Hypersensitivity to paliperidone or risperidone; concurrent use of drugs known to cause QTc prolongation (including quinidine, procainamide, sotalol, amiodarone, chlorpromazine, thioridazine, moxofloxacin); history of congenital QTc prolongation or other cardiac arrhythmias; bradycardia, hypokalemia, hypomagnesemia (↑ risk of QTc prolongation); pre-existing severe GI narrowing (due to nature of tablet formulation); **Lactation:** Discontinue drug or bottle-feed.

Use Cautiously in: Clients with Parkinson's disease or dementia with Lewy bodies (↑ sensitivity to effects of antipsychotics); history of suicide attempts; clients at risk for aspiration pneumonia; history of seizures; conditions that may ↑ body temperature (strenuous exercise, exposure to extreme heat, concurrent anticholinergics, or risk of dehydration); ↑ GI transit time (may ↓ blood levels); may mask symptoms of some drug overdoses, intestinal obstruction, Reye's syndrome, or brain tumor (due to antiemetic effect); diabetes mellitus; severe hepatic impairment; renal impairment (dose reduction recommended if CCr <80 mL/min); *Pregnancy:* Safety not established; use only if maternal benefit outweighs fetal risk.

Adverse Reactions/Side Effects: (CAPITALS indicate life-threatening; <u>underlines</u> indicate most frequent.)

CNS: NEUROLEPTIC MALIGNANT SYNDROME, <u>drowsiness,</u> <u>headache,</u> anxiety, confusion, dizziness, extrapyramidal disorders (dose-related), fatigue, Parkinsonism (dose-related), syncope, TD, weakness. **EENT:** Blurred vision. **Resp:** <u>Dyspnea,</u> cough. **CV:** <u>Palpitations,</u> <u>tachycardia (dose-related),</u> bradycardia, orthostatic hypotension, ↑ QTc interval. **GI:** <u>Abdominal pain,</u> dry mouth, dyspepsia, nausea, swollen tongue. **Endo:** Hyperglycemia. **MS:** Back pain, dystonia. **Neuro:** Akathisia, dyskinesia, tremor (dose-related). **Misc:** Fever.

Interactions: ↑ Risk of CNS depression with other *CNS depressants* including *alcohol, antihistamines, sedatives/hypnotics,* and *opioid analgesics.* May antagonize effects of *levodopa* or other *dopamine agonists.* ↑ Risk of orthostatic hypotension with *antihypertensives, nitrates,* or other *agents that lower blood pressure.*

Dosage: PO (Adults): 6 mg/day; may be titrated as needed (range 3–12 mg/day).

Renal Impairment: PO (Adults): *CCr 50–80 mL/min:* dose should not exceed 6 mg/day; *CCr 10–<50 mL/min:* dose should not exceed 3 mg/day.

Availability: Brand only

Extended-Release Tablets: 3 mg, 6 mg, 9 mg. COST: **$$$$+**

⬡ **Geriatric Considerations:** Not approved for elderly with dementia-related psychosis; ↑ risk for mortality. Dose adjustment with renal impairment.

⬡ **Pediatric/Adolescent Considerations:** Safety not established.

⬡ **Clinical Assessments:** Monitor BP and pulse; ECG with CV symptoms or concern. Monitor for EPS, TD, NMS. (See *Psychotropic Adverse Effects, Basics tab.*) Monitor weight, BMI. FBS, lipids before and during treatment. (See *BMI/Metabolic Syndrome, Tools tab.*) Evaluate mental status, mood, and behavior.

[**Clinical Tips/Alerts:** Do not use with QTc prolongation or other arrhythmias. Monitor for suicidality in high-risk clients. Priapism has been reported.]

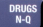

Paroxetine HCl

(par-**ox**-e-teen) Paxil, Paxil CR, **paroxetine mesylate:** Pexeva

Classification: Therapeutic: Antianxiety agents, antidepressants; *Pharmacological:* SSRIs; *Pregnancy Category D*

Indications: **Paxil, Paxil CR, Pexeva:** Major depressive disorder, panic disorder. **Paxil, Pexeva:** OCD, GAD. **Paxil, Paxil CR:** Social anxiety disorder. **Paxil:** Posttraumatic stress disorder (PTSD). **Paxil CR:** PMDD.

Action: Inhibits neuronal reuptake of serotonin in CNS, thus potentiating activity of serotonin; has little effect on norepinephrine or dopamine.

Pharmacokinetics: *Absorption:* Completely absorbed following oral administration. Controlled-release tablets are enteric-coated and control medication release over 4–5 hr. *Distribution:* Widely distributed throughout body fluids and tissues, including CNS; cross placenta and enter breast milk. *Metabolism and Excretion:* Highly metabolized by liver (partly by P450 2D6 enzyme system); 2% excreted unchanged in urine.

Protein Binding: 95%.

T 1/2: 21 hr.

TIME/ACTION PROFILE (antidepressant action)

Route	Onset	Peak	Duration
PO	1–4 wk	Unknown	Unknown

Contraindicated in: Hypersensitivity; concurrent MAOI, thioridazine, or pimozide therapy.

Use Cautiously in: Risk of suicide attempt/ideation esp. during early treatment or dose adjustment); history of seizures; history of bipolar disorder. **Pregnancy:** Use during the first trimester may be associated with an ↑ risk of cardiac malformations: consider fetal risk/maternal benefit; use during third trimester may result in neonatal serotonin syndrome requiring prolonged hospitalization and respiratory and nutritional support. *Lactation:* Safety not established; discontinue drug or bottle-feed.

Adverse Reactions/Side Effects: (CAPITALS indicate life-threatening; underlines indicate most frequent.)

CNS: Anxiety, dizziness, drowsiness, headache, insomnia, weakness, agitation, amnesia, confusion, emotional lability, hangover, impaired concentration, malaise, mental depression, suicidal behavior, syncope. **EENT:** Blurred vision, rhinitis,

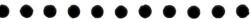

Resp: Cough, pharyngitis, respiratory disorders, yawning. **CV:** Chest pain, edema, hypertension, palpitations, postural hypotension, tachycardia, vasodilation. **GI:** Constipation, diarrhea, dry mouth, nausea, abdominal pain, ↓ appetite, dyspepsia, flatulence, ↑ appetite, taste disturbances, vomiting. **GU:** Ejaculatory disturbance, ↓ libido, genital disorders, urinary disorders, urinary frequency. **Derm:** Sweating, photosensitivity, pruritus, rash. **Metab:** Weight gain, weight loss. **MS:** Back pain, myalgia, myopathy. **Neuro:** Paresthesia, tremor. **Misc:** Chills, fever.

Interactions: Potentially fatal with concurrent *MAOI* therapy. MAOIs should be stopped at least 14 days before paroxetine therapy. Paroxetine should be stopped at least 14 days before MAOI therapy. May ↓ metabolism and ↑ effects of certain *drugs that are metabolized by liver,* including other *antidepressants, phenothiazines, class IC antiarrhythmics, risperidone, atomoxetine, theophylline, procyclidine,* and *quinidine.* Concurrent use should be undertaken with caution. Concurrent use with *pimozide* or *thioridazine* may ↑ risk of QT-interval prolongation and torsades de pointes; concurrent use is contraindicated. *Cimetidine* ↑ blood levels. *Phenobarbital* and *phenytoin* may ↓ effectiveness. Concurrent use with *alcohol* is not recommended. May ↓ effectiveness of *digoxin.* May ↑ risk of *bleeding* with *warfarin, aspirin,* or *NSAIDs.* Concurrent use with *5-HT$_1$ agonists (frovatriptan, naratriptan, rizatriptan, sumatriptan, zolmitriptan), linezolid, lithium,* or *tramadol* may result in ↑ serotonin levels and lead to serotonin syndrome. ***Drug-Natural:*** ↑ Risk of serotonergic side effects including serotonin syndrome with *St. John's wort, SAMe,* and *tryptophan.*

Dosage: **Depression: PO (Adults):** 20 mg as a single dose in the morning; may be ↑ by 10 mg/day at weekly intervals (not to exceed 50 mg/day). *Controlled-release tablets:* 25 mg once daily initially. May ↑ at weekly intervals by 12.5 mg (not to exceed 62.5 mg/day).

PO (Geriatric or Debilitated Clients): 10 mg/day initially; may be slowly ↑ (not to exceed 40 mg/day). *Controlled-release tablets:* 12.5 mg once daily initially; may be slowly ↑ (not to exceed 50 mg/day).

OCD: PO (Adults): 20 mg/day initially; ↑ by 10 mg/day at weekly intervals up to 40 mg (not to exceed 60 mg/day).

Panic Disorder: PO (Adults): 10 mg/day initially; ↑ by 10 mg/day at weekly intervals up to 40 mg (not to exceed 60 mg/day). *Controlled-release tablets:* 12.5 mg/day initially; ↑ by 12.5 mg/day at weekly intervals (not to exceed 75 mg/day).

Social Anxiety Disorder: PO (Adults): 20 mg/day. *Controlled-release tablets:* 12.5 mg/day initially; may ↑ by 12.5 mg/day at weekly intervals (not to exceed 37.5 mg/day).

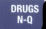

DRUGS N-Q

Paroxetine HCl

GAD: PO (Adults): 20 mg once daily initially; ↑ by 10 mg/day at weekly intervals (not to exceed 50 mg/day).

PTSD: PO (Adults): 20 mg/day initially; may be ↑ by 10 mg/day at weekly intervals (not to exceed 50 mg/day).

PMDD: PO (Adults): *Controlled-release tablets:* 12.5 mg once daily throughout menstrual cycle or during luteal phase of menstrual cycle only; may be ↑ to 25 mg/day after 1 week.

Hepatic Impairment: PO (Adults): *Severe hepatic impairment:* 10 mg/day initially; may be ↑ (not to exceed 40 mg/day). *Controlled-release tablets* 12.5 mg once daily initially; may be slowly ↑ (not to exceed 50 mg/day).

Renal Impairment: PO (Adults): *Severe renal impairment:* 10 mg/day initially; may be slowly ↑ (not to exceed 40 mg/day). *Controlled-release tablets* 12.5 mg once daily initially; may be slowly ↑ (not to exceed 50 mg/day).

Availability (generic available)

Paroxetine Hydrochloride Tablets: 10 mg, 20 mg, 30 mg, 40 mg. COST: *Generic* $.
Paroxetine Hydrochloride Controlled-Release Tablets: 12.5 mg, 25 mg, 37.5 mg. COST: $$. **Paroxetine Hydrochloride Oral Suspension (Orange Flavor):** 10 mg/5 mL. COST: $$$$. **Paroxetine Mesylate Tablets:** 10 mg, 20 mg, 30 mg, 40 mg. COST: $$$$.

● **Geriatric Considerations:** Start at lower initial dose; do not exceed 40 mg/day (controlled release: 50 mg/day). May be sedating (risk for falls). *Caution:* Severe hepatic/renal impairment.

● **Pediatric/Adolescent Considerations:** Paxil was first drug (Seroxat in UK) to result in warnings about suicide in children. Safety has not been established in children, adolescent, young adults. Requires close face-to-face monitoring for suicidality early on in treatment and during dosage adjustments. Studies have shown efficacy for treatment of depression, social anxiety, and OCD in children and adolescents. Monitor closely.

● **Clinical Assessments:** Monitor mental status and for mood changes; reduction or ↑ in anxiety. Monitor weight for gain or loss. Monitor for suicidality early on and during dosage adjustments.

● **Clinical Tips/Alerts:** Paroxetine is good choice for depression associated with anxiety (comorbid anxiety). *Withdrawal syndrome* possible/likely with paroxetine versus other SSRIs: Restlessness, nausea, tingling, and headache. **Must taper slowly.** Potentially fatal with concurrent MAOIs and within 14 days of stopping (see *Serotonin Syndrome, Basics tab*).

Perphenazine

(per-**fen**-a-zeen) Trilafon, *Apo-Perphenazine, PMS Perphenazine*

Classification: *Therapeutic:* Antiemetics, antipsychotics (conventional); *Pharmacological:* Phenothiazines; *Pregnancy Category C*

Indications: Schizophrenia. Nausea and vomiting. **Off-Label Use:** Other psychotic disorders, bipolar disorder. Treatment of intractable hiccups (IV only).

Action: Alters effects of dopamine in CNS. Possesses significant anticholinergic and alpha-adrenergic blocking activity. Blocks dopamine in chemoreceptor trigger zone.

Pharmacokinetics: *Absorption:* Absorption from tablet poor (approximately 20%) and variable; may be better with oral liquid formulations; well absorbed following IM administration. *Distribution:* Widely distributed, high concentrations in CNS; crosses placenta and enters breast milk. *Metabolism and Excretion:* Highly metabolized by liver and GI mucosa; some conversion to active compounds.

Protein Binding: ≥90%.

T $\frac{1}{2}$: 8.4–12.3 hr.

TIME/ACTION PROFILE (PO, IM = antipsychotic effect*; IV = antiemetic effect)

Route	Onset	Peak	Duration
PO	2–6 hr	Unknown	6–12 hr
IM	2–6 hr	Unknown	6–12 hr
IV	Rapid	Unknown	Unknown

*Optimal antipsychotic response may not occur for several weeks

Contraindicated in: Hypersensitivity (cross-sensitivity with other phenothiazines may occur); hypersensitivity to bisulfites (injection only); known alcohol intolerance (concentrate only); angle-closure glaucoma; pre-existing bone marrow depression or blood dyscrasias; severe liver or CV disease; intestinal obstruction. *Lactation:* Discontinue drug or bottle-feed.

Use Cautiously in: Geriatric, emaciated, or debilitated clients (one half to one third of usual initial dose recommended); diabetes mellitus; respiratory disease; prostatic hyperplasia; CNS tumors; history of seizure disorder. *Pregnancy:* Safety not established.

Adverse Reactions/Side Effects: (CAPITALS indicate life-threatening; underlines indicate most frequent.)

CNS: NEUROLEPTIC MALIGNANT SYNDROME, extrapyramidal reactions, sedation, tardive dyskinesia. **EENT:** Blurred vision, dry eyes, lens opacities. **CV:** Hypotension, tachycardia. **GI:** Constipation, dry mouth, anorexia, ileus, weight gain. **GU:** Discoloration of urine, urinary retention. **Derm:** Photosensitivity, pigment changes, rashes. **Endo:** Galactorrhea, amenorrhea. **Hemat:** AGRANULOCYTOSIS, leukopenia. **Metab:** Hyperthermia. **Misc:** Allergic reactions.

Interactions: Additive hypotension with *antihypertensives;* acute ingestion of *alcohol,* or *nitrates.* Additive CNS depression with *MAOIs* or other *CNS depressants,* including alcohol, antihistamines, opioid analgesics, *sedative/hypnotics,* and general anesthetics. Additive anticholinergic effects with other *drugs possessing anticholinergic properties,* including antihistamines, antidepressants, atropine, disopyramide, haloperidol, and other phenothiazines. Hypotension and tachycardia may occur with epinephrine. ↑ Risk of agranulocytosis with other agents that cause bone-marrow suppression, including antithyroid agents. ↑ Risk of extrapyramidal reactions with *lithium.* May mask *lithium* toxicity. Antacids or *lithium* may ↑ absorption of perphenazine. May ↑ antiparkinson effect of *levodopa* or *bromocriptine.* **Drug-Natural:** ↑ Anticholinergic effects with *angel's trumpet, jimson weed,* and *scopola.*

Dosage: **PO (Adults):** *Schizophrenia:* 2–16 mg two to four times daily (not to exceed 64 mg/day). **IM (Adults):** *Psychoses:* 5–10 mg initially; may repeat every 6 hr (not to exceed 15–30 mg/day).

Availability (generic available)
Tablets: 2 mg, 4 mg, 8 mg, 16 mg. COST: **$.** **Syrup:** Canadian: 2 mg/5 mL. **Oral Concentrate:** 16 mg/5 mL. **Injection:** 5 mg/mL in 1-mL ampules. *In Combination with:* Amitriptyline (Etrafon, Triavil).

● **Geriatric Considerations:** Caution because of sedation and anticholinergic effects; additive with other CNS medications and anticholinergics. ↑ Risk of mortality in elderly with dementia-related psychosis.
● **Pediatric/Adolescent Considerations:** Safety not established. No indications for use.
● **Clinical Assessments:** Monitor CBC, LFT, and eye examinations periodically. Agranulocytosis may begin 4–10 weeks after starting treatment. Monitor for mental status; positive and negative symptoms of schizophrenia. Monitor for EPS, TD, NMS. (See *Psychotropic Adverse Effects, Basics tab.*) Monitor weight, BMI, FBS, and lipids. (See *BMI/Metabolic Syndrome, Tools tab.*)

[**Clinical Tips/Alerts:** Atypical should be first-line treatment; perphenazine is sedating and can cause weight gain. Caution with additive effects of alcohol, sedatives, and antihistamines.]

Phenelzine

(**fen**-el-zeen) Nardil

Classification: *Therapeutic:* Antidepressants; *Pharmacological:* MAOI; *Pregnancy Category C*

Indications: Treatment of neurotic or atypical depression (usually reserved for clients who do not tolerate or respond to other modes of therapy [e.g., tricyclic antidepressants, SSRIs, SSNRIs, or electroconvulsive therapy]).

Action: Inhibits enzyme monoamine oxidase, resulting in accumulation of neurotransmitters (dopamine, epinephrine, norepinephrine, and serotonin).

Pharmacokinetics: *Absorption:* Well absorbed from GI tract.

Distribution: Crosses placenta and probably enters breast milk. *Metabolism* and *Excretion* : Metabolized by liver; excreted in urine as metabolites and unchanged drug.

T $^1/_2$: 12 hr.

TIME/ACTION PROFILE (antidepressant effect)

Route	Onset	Peak	Duration
PO	2–4 wk	3–6 wk	2 wk

Contraindicated in: *Lactation.* Hypersensitivity; liver disease; severe renal disease; pheochromocytoma; heart failure; clients undergoing elective surgery requiring general anesthesia (should be discontinued at least 10 days before surgery); excessive consumption of caffeine; concurrent use of meperidine, SSRI antidepressants, SNRI antidepressants, tricyclic antidepressants, tetracyclic antidepressants, nefazodone, trazodone, procarbazine, selegiline, linezolid, carbamazepine, cyclobenzaprine, bupropion, buspirone, sympathomimetics, other MAOIs, dextromethorphan, narcotics, alcohol, general anesthetics, diuretics, or tryptophan; concurrent use of foods containing high concentrations of tyramine (*see MAOI diet; Tools tab*).

Use Cautiously in: Clients who may be suicidal or have a history of drug dependency; schizophrenia; bipolar disorder; seizure disorders; diabetes (↑ risk of hypoglycemia); *Pregnancy:* Safety not established.

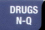

DRUGS N-Q

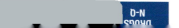

DRUGS
N-Q

Adverse Reactions/Side Effects: (CAPITALS indicate life-threatening; underlines indicate most frequent.)

CNS: SEIZURES, dizziness, drowsiness, fatigue, headache, hyperreflexia, insomnia, tremor, twitching, weakness, euphoria, paresthesia, restlessness. **EENT:** Blurred vision, glaucoma, nystagmus. **CV:** HYPERTENSIVE CRISIS, edema, orthostatic hypotension. **GI:** Constipation, dry mouth, abdominal pain, liver function test elevation, nausea, vomiting. **GU:** Sexual dysfunction, urinary retention. **Derm:** Pruritus, rashes. **F and E:** Hypernatremia. **Endo:** Weight gain.

Interactions: Potentially fatal adverse reactions may occur with concurrent use of other antidepressants, carbamazepine, cyclobenzaprine, sibutramine, procarbazine, or *selegiline.* Hypertensive crisis may occur with amphetamines, methyldopa, levodopa, dopamine, epinephrine, norepinephrine, reserpine, methylphenidate, or vasoconstrictors. Hypertension or hypotension, coma, seizures, respiratory depression, and death may occur with meperidine (avoid using within 2–3 wk of MAOI therapy). Concurrent use with dextromethorphan may produce psychosis or bizarre behavior. Hypertension may occur with concurrent use of buspirone; avoid using within 2 wk of each other. Additive hypotension may occur with antihypertensives, spinal anesthesia, opioids, or barbiturates. Additive hypoglycemia may occur with insulins or oral hypoglycemic agents. Risk of seizures may be ↑ with tramadol. **Drug-Natural:** Serious, potentially fatal adverse effects (serotonin syndrome) may occur with concurrent use of St. John's wort and SAMe. Hypertensive crises may occur with large amounts of caffeine-containing herbs (cola nut, guarana, or maté). Insomnia, headache, tremor, and hypomania may occur with ginseng. Hypertensive crises, disorientation, and memory impairment may occur with tryptophan or supplements containing tyrosine or phenylalanine. **Drug-Food:** Hypertensive crisis may occur with ingestion of foods containing high concentrations of tyramine (see MAOI diet, Tools tab). Consumption of foods or beverages with high caffeine content ↑ risk of hypertension and arrhythmias.

Dosage: PO (Adults): 15 mg three times daily; ↑ to 60–90 mg/day in divided doses; after maximal benefit achieved, gradually reduce to smallest effective dose (15 mg/day or every other day).

Availability (generic available)
Tablets: 15 mg. COST: **$$**

● **Geriatric Considerations:** Elderly have greater sensitivity to adverse effects; evaluate for ability to follow diet.

- **Pediatric/Adolescent Considerations:** Safety and effectiveness not established. Monitor face to face for suicidality early in treatment and during dosage adjustments.
- **Substance Abuse Considerations:** Do not use MAOIs with substance abuse clients unable to abstain, because of possible serious interactions.

Clinical Assessments: Assess/monitor for mood improvement, suicidality; *monitor BP* and *pulse before* and *during treatment*; weight and BMI before and during treatment. Other tests: FBS, lipids. (See *BMI/Metabolic Syndrome, Tools tab*.)

> **Clinical Tips/Alerts:** Potentially fatal reactions (serotonin syndrome) with concurrent use of other *antidepressants (SSRIs, SNRIs, bupropion, tricyclics, tetracyclics, nefazodone, trazodone), carbamazepine, cyclobenzaprine, ibutramine, procarbazine,* or *selegiline*). Avoid using within at least 2 wk of each other (wait 5 wk from end of *fluoxetine* therapy). (See *serotonin syndrome in Basics tab*.) Client **must be willing to follow MAOI (tyramine-restricted) diet** to avoid hypertensive crisis (*emergency*). (See *MAOI Diet, Tools tab*.) Avoid *meperidine.* Although not a first-line treatment, should be considered for treatment-resistant depression. Associated with weight gain and sedation.

Pimozide

(**pi**-mo-zide) Orap

Classification: *Therapeutic:* Antipsychotics (conventional); *Pregnancy Category C*

Indications: Suppression of motor and vocal tics in Tourette's disorder with severe, compromising symptoms in clients with an unfavorable response to haloperidol. Second-line treatment after failure with atypical antipsychotics. **Off-Label Use:** Psychotic disorders that fail to respond to standard treatment.

Action: Blocks dopamine receptors in CNS. ↑ Brain turnover of dopamine, blocks calcium channels, and may antagonize opiate receptors.

Pharmacokinetics: *Absorption:* 50% absorbed following oral administration. *Distribution:* Unknown. *Metabolism* and *Excretion:* Undergoes extensive first-pass hepatic metabolism, at least partly by P450 3A4 (CYP3A4) and CYP1A2 enzyme systems. Some metabolites have CNS activity.

T $\frac{1}{2}$: 29–111 hr.

TIME/ACTION PROFILE (blood levels)

Route	Onset	Peak	Duration
PO	Unknown	6–8 hr	Unknown

Contraindicated in: Hypersensitivity (cross-sensitivity with other antipsychotics may occur); concurrent use of agents that may be causing the motor and vocal tics; congenital long QT syndrome (↑ risk of serious arrhythmias); recent MI, heart failure; concurrent use of agents that prolong QT interval, including dofetilide, sotalol, quinidine, other class IA or III antiarrhythmics, thioridazine, chlorpromazine, droperidol, sparfloxacin, moxifloxacin, mefloquine, pentamidine, arsenic trioxide, levomethadyl acetate, dolasetron, tacrolimus, ziprasidone, clarithromycin, and azithromycin (↑ risk of serious arrhythmias); concurrent use of CYP3A4 enzyme inhibitors, including erythromycin, clarithromycin, azithromycin, itraconazole, ketoconazole, saquinavir, indinavir, nelfinavir, nefazodone, zileuton, and fluvoxamine (↑ risk of serious arrhythmias); CNS depression or comatose state; motor or vocal tics not caused by Tourette's disorder; hypokalemia, hypomagnesemia (↑ risk of serious arrhythmias).

Use Cautiously in: History of breast cancer; angle-closure glaucoma; history of paralytic ileus; hepatic or renal impairment; prostatic hyperplasia; history of seizures (threshold may be lowered); hypokalemia (↑ risk of arrhythmias). **Lactation:** Safety not established, discontinue drug or bottle-feed. **Pregnancy:** Safety not established.

Adverse Reactions/Side Effects: (CAPITALS indicate life-threatening; underlines indicate most frequent.)
CNS: NEUROLEPTIC MALIGNANT SYNDROME, mood/behavior effects, weakness, drowsiness. **EENT:** Blurred vision, dry eyes. **CV:** ARRHYTHMIAS (PROLONGED QT INTERVAL), hypotension. **GI:** Constipation, dry mouth, ↑ appetite, nausea, vomiting, weight loss. **GU:** Libido, erectile dysfunction. **Derm:** Skin discoloration. **Endo:** Galactorrhea (women). **Hemat:** Blood dyscrasias. **Neuro:** Akathisia, parkinsonism, dystonic reactions, tardive dyskinesia, akinesia.

Interactions: Concurrent use of macrolide anti-infectives (erythromycin, clarithromycin, azithromycin), dofetilide, sotalol, quinidine, other class IA or III antiarrhythmics, thioridazine, chlorpromazine, droperidol, sparfloxacin, gemifloxacin, moxifloxacin, mefloquine, pentamidine, arsenic trioxide, dolasetron, tacrolimus, and ziprasidone ↑ risk of serious ventricular arrhythmias and should be avoided; similar effects may occur with tricyclic antidepressants, disopyramide, and procainamide.

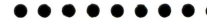

Blood levels and risk of cardiac arrhythmias are ↑ by concurrent use of *ritonavir;* concurrent use is contraindicated. Metabolism of pimozide may be impaired by azole antifungals; concurrent use of *intraconazole, fluvoxamine,* and *ketoconazole* is contraindicated. ↑ Risk of CNS depression with *alcohol* or other *CNS depressants. Amphetamines, methylphenidate,* or *pemoline* may provoke tics that cannot be treated with pimozide; discontinue these before initiating therapy with pimozide. Block effects of *amphetamines.* Concurrent use with *MAOIs* ↑ risk of sedative, hypotensive, and anticholinergic adverse reactions. Concurrent use with *fluoxetine* may result in bradycardia. **Drug-Natural:** Concomitant use of *kava, valerian,* or *chamomile* can ↑ CNS depression. *St. John's wort* may affect pimozide levels and effectiveness; avoid concurrent use. **Drug-Food:** *Grapefruit juice* ↑ risks of arrythmias.

Dosage: **Tourette's Disorder: PO (Adults):** 1–2 mg/day in divided doses, may be ↑ gradually as needed and tolerated up to 0.2 mg/kg/day or 10 mg/day, whichever is less.

PO (Children >12 yr): 0.05 mg/kg/day as a single bedtime dose, may be ↑ every third day as needed and tolerated up to 0.2 mg/kg/day or 10 mg/day, whichever is less.

PO (Geriatric Clients): Use lower initial doses and more gradual titration.

Psychotic Disorders (off label)

PO (Adults): 2–4 mg/day as a single morning dose; may be ↑ by 2–4 mg/day at weekly intervals as needed and tolerated (usual dose is 6 mg/day, range 2–12 mg/day); up to 0.3 mg/kg/day or 20 mg/day, whichever is less.

Availability

Tablets: Canadian: 1 mg, 2 mg. COST: **$–$$.** Canadian: 4 mg, Canadian: 10 mg.

- **Geriatric Considerations:** ↑ Sensitivity to side effects. ↑ Risk of mortality in elderly with dementia-related psychosis.
- **Pediatric/Adolescent Considerations:** ↑ Sensitivity to side effects.
- **Clinical Assessments:** ECG before and during treatment. Assess mental status and tic frequency. Monitor weight, BMI, FBS, and lipids. (See *BMI/Metabolic Syndrome, Tools tab.*) Assess for EPS, TD, and NMS. (See *Psychotropic Adverse Effects, Basics tab.*)

[Clinical Tips/Alerts: Do not use with long QT syndrome, MI, heart failure; ↑ risk of life-threatening arrhythmias. (See also preceding Interactions.) Not a first-line treatment for psychosis or Tourette's disorder. **]**

 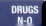

Propranolol

(proe-**pran**-oh-lol) Inderal, Inderal LA, InnoPran XL, Apo-Propranolol, Betachron E-R, Novopranol, pms Propranolol

Classification: Therapeutic: Antianginals, antiarrhythmics (class II), antihypertensives, vascular headache suppressants; Pharmacological: Beta blockers; Pregnancy Category C

Indications: Management of hypertension, angina, arrhythmias, hypertrophic cardiomyopathy, thyrotoxicosis, essential tremors, pheochromocytoma. Also used in prevention and management of MI and prevention of vascular headaches. **Off-Label Use:** Used to manage alcohol withdrawal, aggressive behavior, antipsychotic-associated akathisia, situational anxiety, and esophageal varices, PTSD (ongoing clinical trials at National Institute for Mental Health [NIMH]).

Action: Blocks stimulation of beta-1 (myocardial) and beta-2 (pulmonary, vascular, and uterine) adrenergic receptor sites.

Pharmacokinetics: Absorption: Well absorbed but undergoes extensive first-pass hepatic metabolism. Distribution: Moderate CNS penetration. Crosses placenta; enters breast milk. Metabolism and Excretion: Almost completely metabolized by liver.

Protein Binding: 93%.

T 1/2: 3.4–6 hr.

TIME/ACTION PROFILE (CV effects)

Route	Onset	Peak	Duration
PO	30 min	60–90 min*	6–12 hr
PO-ER	Unknown	6 hr	24 hr
IV	immediate	1 min	4–6 hr

*Following single dose, full effect not seen until several weeks of therapy

Contraindicated in: Uncompensated CHF; pulmonary edema; cardiogenic shock; bradycardia or heart block.

Use Cautiously in: Renal or hepatic impairment; pulmonary disease (including asthma); diabetes mellitus (may mask signs of hypoglycemia); thyrotoxicosis (may mask symptoms); history of severe allergic reactions (may ↑ intensity of response). **Pregnancy:** Crosses placenta and may cause fetal/neonatal bradycardia, hypotension, hypoglycemia, or respiratory depression. May also ↑ blood supply to placenta.

↑ risk for premature birth or fetal death, and cause intrauterine growth retardation. May ↑ risk of cardiac and pulmonary complications in infant during neonatal time frame. *Lactation:* Appears in breast milk; use formula if propranolol must be taken.

Adverse Reactions/Side Effects: (CAPITALS indicate life-threatening; underlines indicate most frequent.)

CNS: Fatigue, weakness, anxiety, dizziness, drowsiness, insomnia, memory loss, mental depression, mental status changes, nervousness, nightmares. **EENT:** Blurred vision, dry eyes, nasal stuffiness. **Resp:** Bronchospasm, wheezing. **CV:** ARRHYTHMIAS, BRADYCARDIA, CHF, PULMONARY EDEMA, orthostatic hypotension, peripheral vasoconstriction. **GI:** Constipation, diarrhea, nausea. **GU:** Erectile dysfunction, ↓ libido. **Derm:** Itching, rashes. **Endo:** Hyperglycemia, hypoglycemia (↑ in children). **MS:** Arthralgia, back pain, muscle cramps. **Neuro:** Paresthesia. **Misc:** Drug-induced lupus syndrome.

Interactions: *General anesthesia, IV phenytoin,* and *verapamil* may cause additive myocardial depression. Additive bradycardia may occur with *digoxin.* Additive hypotension may occur with other *antihypertensives,* acute ingestion of *alcohol,* or *nitrates.* Concurrent use with *amphetamines, cocaine, ephedrine, epinephrine, norepinephrine, phenylephrine,* or *pseudoephedrine* may result in unopposed alpha-adrenergic stimulation (excessive hypertension, bradycardia). Concurrent *thyroid* administration may ↓ effectiveness. May alter effectiveness of *insulin* or *oral hypoglycemics* (dose adjustments may be necessary). May ↓ effectiveness *of beta-adrenergic bronchodilators* and *theophylline.* May ↓ beneficial beta CV effects of *dopamine* or *dobutamine. Use cautiously within 14 days of MAOI therapy (may result in hypertension). Cimetidine* may ↑ blood levels and toxicity. Concurrent *NSAIDs* may ↓ antihypertensive action. *Smoking* ↑ metabolism and ↓ effects; smoking cessation may ↑ effects.

Dosage: PO (Adults): *Management of Tremor:* 40 mg twice daily; may be ↑ up to 120 mg/day (up to 320 mg has been used).

Availability (generic available)

Oral Solution: 4 mg/mL, 8 mg/mL. COST: *Generic* **$**. Tablets: 10 mg, 20 mg, 40 mg, 60 mg, 80 mg. COST: *Generic* **$**. Sustained-Release Capsules (Inderal LA): 60 mg, 80 mg, 120 mg, 160 mg. COST: $$–$$$. **Extended-Release Capsules:** 60 mg, 80 mg, 120 mg, 160 mg. COST: *Generic* **$$–$$$**. Injection: 1 mg/mL. *In Combination With:* Hydrochlorothiazide (Inderide).

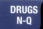

● ● ● ● ● ● ● ● ● ●

Contraindicated in: Hypersensitivity. **Lactation:** Discontinue drug or bottle-feed. **Use Cautiously in:** CV disease, cerebrovascular disease, dehydration, or hypovolemia (↑ risk of hypotension); history of seizures; Alzheimer's dementia;

TIME/ACTION PROFILE (antipsychotic effects)

Route	Onset	Peak	Duration
PO	Unknown	Unknown	8–12 hr
PO-XR	Unknown	Unknown	Unknown

$T\,{1/2}$: 6 hr.

Pharmacokinetics: Absorption: Well absorbed after oral administration. **Distribution:** Widely distributed. **Metabolism and Excretion:** Extensively metabolized by liver (mostly by P450 CYP3A4 enzyme system); <1% excreted unchanged in the urine.

Action: Probably acts by serving as antagonist of dopamine and serotonin. Also antagonizes histamine H_1 receptors and alpha-1 adrenergic receptors.

Indications: Schizophrenia. Depressive episodes with bipolar disorder. Bipolar mania associated with bipolar I as monotherapy or with lithium or divalproex.

Classification: Therapeutic: Antipsychotics, mood stabilizers; **Pregnancy Category C**

(kwet-**eye**-a-peen) Seroquel, Seroquel XR

Quetiapine

with the physical symptoms of panic disorder, phobias (e.g., palpitations).
use concurrently with MAOI or within 14 days of MAOI. Propranolol may help
Bradycardia, severe dizziness or drowsiness, dyspnea, and seizures. Do not
Withdrawal of drug requires slow taper at least over 2 weeks. Overdose signs:
● **Clinical Tips/Alerts:** Caution with diabetics (may ↑ or ↓ blood sugar).

Abrupt withdrawal of propranolol can be life-threatening (arrhythmias, MI).
● **Clinical Assessments:** Monitor BP and pulse before and during treatment.
Monitor BP and pulse before and during treatment. Monitor for hypotension and/or rebound hypertension. Monitor renal insufficiency.
ods of fasting such as before surgery, during prolonged exertion, or with coexist-
● **Pediatric/Adolescent Considerations:** ↑ Risk of hypoglycemia, esp. during peri-
reduction and careful titration recommended.
● **Geriatric Considerations:** ↑ Sensitivity to all beta blockers; initial dose

hypothyroidism (may be exacerbated); history of suicide attempt. *Pregnancy:* Safety not established.

Adverse Reactions/Side Effects: (CAPITALS indicate life-threatening; <u>underlines</u> indicate most frequent.)

CNS: NEUROLEPTIC MALIGNANT SYNDROME, SEIZURES, <u>dizziness,</u> cognitive impairment, extrapyramidal symptoms, sedation, TD. **EENT:** Ear pain, rhinitis, pharyngitis. **Resp:** Cough, dyspnea. **CV:** Palpitations, peripheral edema, postural hypotension. **GI:** Anorexia, constipation, dry mouth, dyspepsia. **Derm:** Sweating. **Hemat:** Leukopenia. **Metab:** <u>Weight gain.</u> **Misc:** Flu-like syndrome.

Interactions: ↑ CNS depression may occur with *alcohol, antihistamines, opioid analgesics,* and *sedative/hypnotics.* ↑ Risk of hypotension with acute ingestion of *alcohol* or *antihypertensives. Phenytoin* and *thioridazine* ↑ clearance and ↓ effectiveness of quetiapine (dose change may be necessary); similar effects may occur with *carbamazepine, barbiturates, rifampin,* or *corticosteroids.* Effects may be ↑ by *ketoconazole, itraconazole, fluconazole,* or *erythromycin,* as well as by other *agents that inhibit it the cytochrome P450 CYP3A4 enzyme.*

Dosage: PO (Adults): *Schizophrenia:* 25 mg twice daily initially, ↑ by 25–50 mg two to three times daily over 3 days, up to 300–400 mg/day in two to three divided doses by the fourth day (not to exceed 800 mg/day); or 300 mg once daily as XR tablets, ↑ by 300 mg/day, up to 400–800 mg/day (not to exceed 800 mg/day). **Elderly clients** or **clients with hepatic impairment** should be started on immediate-release product and converted to XR product once effective dose is reached. *Bipolar Mania:* 100 mg/day in two divided doses on first day, ↑ dose by 100 mg/day up to 400 mg/day by fourth day, then may ↑ in 200 mg/day increments up to 800 mg/day on sixth day if required.

Depressive Bipolar Disorder: Once daily at bedtime to reach 300 mg by fourth day with the following schedule: day 1: 50 mg; day 2: 100 mg; day 3: 200 mg; day 4: 300 mg. *Bipolar Manic Disorder:* Initially 50 mg twice daily, increasing to 400 mg/day by fourth day in increments of up to 100 mg/day in divided doses. Further dose adjustments up to 800 mg/day should be made in increments no greater than 200 mg/day in divided doses.

Availability: Brand only

Tablets: 25 mg, 50 mg, 100 mg, 200 mg, 300 mg, 400 mg. COST: **$$$$. Extended-Release Tablets:** 200 mg, 300 mg, 400 mg. COST: **$$$$.**

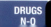

**DRUGS
N–O**

- **Geriatric Considerations:** Requires initial dose reduction; start with immediate-release tablet (see Dosage); contraindicated in elderly with dementia-related psychosis because of ↑ risk of mortality.
- **Pediatric/Adolescent Considerations:** Safety not established; weigh benefits versus risks; monitor face to face for mood improvement with depression and ↑ suicidality early in treatment and during dosage adjustments. Has been used off label for mood disorders, agitation, and behavioral disturbances in children and adolescents. Monitor closely.
- **Clinical Assessments:** Monitor mental status, mood, and behavior. Assess for and monitor for suicidality. Monitor for EPS, TD, and NMS. (See *Psychotropic Adverse Effects, Basics tab.*) Monitor weight, BMI, waist circumference, FBS, and lipids before and during treatment. (See *BMI/Metabolic Syndrome, Tools tab.*) LFTs for ↑ in AST and ALT and eye examinations periodically.

Clinical Tips/Alerts: Weight gain and sedation common; be aware of life-threatening diabetic ketoacidosis (can result in coma and death). Monitor for suicidality.

Psychotropic Drugs R–Z

Ramelteon

(ra-**mel**-tee-on) Rozerem

Classification: *Therapeutic:* Sedatives/hypnotics; *Pharmacological:* Melatonin receptor agonists; *Pregnancy Category C*

Indications: Treatment of insomnia characterized by difficulty falling asleep (sleep onset).

Action: Activates melatonin receptors, which promote maintenance of circadian rhythm, part of the sleep-wake cycle.

Pharmacokinetics: *Absorption:* Well absorbed (84%) but bioavailability low (1.8%) due to extensive first-pass liver metabolism. Absorption ↑ by high-fat meal.

Distribution: Widely distributed to body tissues.

Metabolism and Excretion: Extensively metabolized by liver; mainly by CYP1A2 enzyme system. Metabolites excreted mostly in urine (80%); 4% excreted in feces.

T $\frac{1}{2}$: 1–2.6 hr.

TIME/ACTION PROFILE (blood levels)

Route	Onset	Peak	Duration
PO	Rapid	30–90 min	Unknown

Contraindicated in: *Lactation.* Hypersensitivity; severe hepatic impairment; concurrent fluvoxamine; **Pedi:** Safety not established.

Use Cautiously in: Depression or history of suicidal ideation; moderate hepatic impairment; concurrent use of CYP3A4 inhibitors, such as ketoconazole; concurrent use of CYP2C9 inhibitors, such as fluconazole. ***Pregnancy:*** Use only if maternal benefit outweighs fetal risk.

Adverse Reactions/Side Effects: (CAPITALS indicate life-threatening; <u>underlines</u> indicate most frequent.)

CNS: Abnormal thinking, behavior changes, dizziness, fatigue, hallucinations, headache, insomnia (worsened), sleep-driving. **GI:** Nausea. **Endo:** ↑ Prolactin levels, ↓ Testosterone levels. **MISC:** ANAPHYLACTIC REACTION.

Interactions: Blood levels and effects are ↑ by *fluvoxamine*, potent inhibitor of CYP1A2 enzyme system; *concurrent use contraindicated.* Levels and effects may be

↑ by *rifampin*, an inducer of CYP enzymes. Concurrent use of CYP3A4 inhibitors, such as *ketoconazole*, may ↑ levels and effects; use cautiously. Concurrent use of CYP2C9 inhibitors, such as *fluconazole*, may ↑ levels and effects; use cautiously. ↑ Risk of excessive CNS depression with other CNS depressants including *alcohol, benzodiazepines, opioids,* and other *sedatives/hypnotics*.

Dosage: PO (Adults): 8 mg within 30 min of going to bed.

Availability: Brand only
Tablets: 8 mg. COST: **$$**

● **Geriatric Considerations:** No overall differences in safety or efficacy were observed between elderly and younger adults. Caution with hepatic disease, and be aware of sedation (take within 30 minutes of bedtime and be prepared for sleep).

● **Pediatric/Adolescent Considerations:** Safety not established. No current indications.

● **Clinical Assessments:** Assess sleep patterns before and during treatment.

● **Clinical Tips/Alerts:** Clients have been known to perform activities (cook/eat/drive) *while asleep* (complex sleep-related behaviors) and *serious allergic reactions* have happened (swelling of tongue/throat, difficulty breathing) requiring emergency care. If angioedema develops, seek emergency treatment, and do not use drug again. Take within 30 minutes of bedtime. (See drug interactions for cautions and contraindications).

Risperidone

(riss-**per**-i-done) Risperdal, Risperdal M-TAB, Risperdal Consta

Classification: *Therapeutic:* Antipsychotics, mood stabilizers; *Pharmacological:* Benzisoxazoles; *Pregnancy Category C*

Indications: Schizophrenia in adults and adolescents 13–17 yr. Bipolar mania (oral only) in adults and children 10–17 yr; can be used with lithium or valproate (adults only) in adults with autistic disorder in children 5–16 yr.

Action: May act by antagonizing dopamine and serotonin in CNS.

Pharmacokinetics: *Absorption:* 70% after administration of tablets, solution, or orally disintegrating tablets. Following IM administration, small initial release of drug, followed by 3–week lag; rest of release starts at 3 weeks and lasts 4–6 weeks.

Distribution: Unknown.

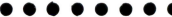

Metabolism and Excretion: Extensively metabolized by liver. Metabolism genetically determined; extensive metabolizers (most clients) convert risperidone to 9-hydroxyrisperidone rapidly. Poor metabolizers (6%–8% of whites) convert more slowly. The 9-hydroxyrisperidone is an antipsychotic compound. Risperidone and its active metabolite are eliminated renally.

T $^1/_2$: *Extensive metabolizers:* 3 hr for risperidone, 21 hr for 9-hydroxyrisperidone. *Poor metabolizers:* 20 hr for risperidone, 30 hr for 9-hydroxyrisperidone.

TIME/ACTION PROFILE (clinical effects)

Route	Onset	Peak	Duration
PO	1–2 wk	Unknown	Up to 6 wk*
IM	3 wk	4–6 wk	Up to 6 wk*

*After discontinuation.

Contraindicated in: Hypersensitivity. *Lactation:* Discontinue drug or bottle-feed.
Use Cautiously in: Debilitated clients, clients with renal or hepatic impairment (initial dose reduction recommended); underlying CV disease (may be more prone to arrhythmias and hypotension); history of seizures; history of suicide attempt or drug abuse; diabetes or risk factors for diabetes (may worsen glucose control); clients at risk for aspiration. *Pregnancy:* Safety not established.
Adverse Reactions/Side Effects: (CAPITALS indicate life-threatening; underlines indicate most frequent.)
CNS: NMS, aggressive behavior, dizziness, extrapyramidal reactions, headache, ↑ dreams, ↑ sleep duration, insomnia, sedation, fatigue, impaired temperature regulation, nervousness, tardive dyskinesia (TD). **EENT:** Pharyngitis, rhinitis, visual disturbances. **Resp:** Cough, dyspnea. **CV:** Arrhythmias, orthostatic hypotension, tachycardia. **GI:** Constipation, diarrhea, dry mouth, nausea, abdominal pain, anorexia, dyspepsia, ↑ salivation, vomiting, weight gain, weight loss, polydipsia. **GU:** ↓ libido, dysmenorrhea/menorrhagia, difficulty urinating, polyuria. **Derm:** Itching/skin rash, dry skin, ↑ pigmentation, ↑ sweating, photosensitivity, seborrhea. **Endo:** Galactorrhea, hyperglycemia. **MS:** Arthralgia, back pain.
Interactions: May ↓ antiparkinsonian effects of *levodopa* or other *dopamine agonists. Carbamazepine, phenytoin, rifampin, phenobarbital,* and *other enzyme inducers* ↑ metabolism and may ↓ effectiveness; dose adjustments may be necessary. *Fluoxetine* and *paroxetine* ↑ blood levels and may ↑ effects; dose adjustments may

be necessary. *Clozapine* ↑ metabolism and may ↑ effects of risperidone. ↑ CNS depression may occur with other CNS depressants, including alcohol, antihistamines, *sedatives/hypnotics*, or opioid analgesics. **Drug-Natural:** Kava, valerian, or *chamomile* can ↓ CNS depression.

Dosage: Schizophrenia: PO (Adults): 1 mg twice daily, ↑ by 1–2 mg/day no more frequently than every 24 hr to 4–8 mg daily. **PO (Children 13–17 yr):** 0.5 mg once daily, ↑ by 0.5–1 mg no more frequently than every 24 hr to 3 mg daily. **IM (Adults):** 25 mg every 2 weeks; some clients may require larger dose of 37.5 or 50 mg every 2 weeks. **Bipolar Mania: PO (Adults):** 2–3 mg/day as a single daily dose, dose may be ↑ at 24-hr intervals by 1 mg (range 1–5 mg/day). **PO (Children 13–17 yrs):** 0.5 mg once daily, ↑ by 0.5–1 mg no more frequently than every 24 hr to 2.5 mg daily. May administer half the daily dose twice daily if drowsiness persists. **PO (Geriatric or Debilitated Clients):** Start with 0.5 mg twice daily, ↑ by 0.5 mg twice daily, up to 1.5 mg twice daily; then ↑ at weekly intervals if necessary. May also be given as a single daily dose after initial titration.

Irritability Associated With Autistic Disorder: PO (Children 5–16 yr weighing <20 kg): 0.25 mg/day initially. After at least 4 days of therapy may ↑ to 0.50 mg/day. Dose ↑ in increments of 0.25 mg/day may be considered at intervals of 2 weeks or longer. May be single or divided dose. **PO (Children 5–16 yr weighing >20 kg):** 0.50 mg/day initially. After at least 4 days of therapy may ↑ to 1 mg/day. Dose ↑ in increments of 0.5 mg/day may be considered at intervals of 2 weeks or longer. May be single or divided dose.

Renal Impairment/Hepatic Impairment: PO (Adults): Start with 0.5 mg twice daily, ↑ by 0.5 mg twice daily, up to 1.5 mg twice daily; then ↑ at weekly intervals if necessary. May also be given as single daily dose after initial titration.

Availability (generic tablets available)

Tablets: 0.25 mg, 0.5 mg, 1 mg, 2 mg, 3 mg, 4 mg. COST: **$$$$**. **Orally Disintegrating Tablets (Risperdal M-Tabs):** 0.5 mg, 1 mg, 2 mg, 3 mg, 4 mg. COST: **$$$$**. **Oral Solution:** 1 mg/mL in 30-mL bottles. COST: **$$–$$$$**. **Microspheres for Injection (Risperdal Consta)** (requires specific diluent for suspension): 12.5 mg/vial kit, 25 mg/vial kit, 37.5 mg/vial kit, 50 mg/vial kit. COST: **$$$$**.

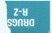

● **Geriatric Considerations:** Initial dose reduction (start 0.5 mg twice/day). Cerebrovascular adverse events, including stroke, reported in elderly who have dementia-related psychosis, *with* ↑ risk for mortality. Not approved for clients with dementia-related psychosis.

- **Pediatric/Adolescent Considerations:** Safety not established. Monitor for sedation, EPS, lactation, gynecomastia. Monitor closely; also monitor closely for suicidality.
- **Clinical Assessments:** Monitor weight, BMI, FBS, Hgb A1C, and cholesterol before and during prescription. (See *BMI/Metabolic Syndrome, Tools tab.*) CBC, LFTs, and eye examinations periodically. Monitor for EPS, TD (rare), and NMS. (See *Psychotropic Adverse Effects, Basics tab.*) Evaluate mental status, mood, and behavior.

Clinical Tips/Alerts: EPS more likely (dose-dependent): ↑ Risk of EPS with doses >6 mg/day and not more efficacious. Potentially less weight gain/diabetes than olanzapine. Titrate slowly at no more than 1–2 mg/day every 24 hr or longer. Convenient *M-Tab* rapidly disintegrates in mouth without water. *Consta* is only long-acting (given deep IM) atypical antipsychotic (injection every 2 weeks). *Consta:* Oral risperidone or other antipsychotic given for 3 weeks after initial injection, then discontinued. If unsure of reaction to risperidone or hepatic impairment, test dose (12.5 mg) rather than give full initial dose. Monitor for suicidality in high-risk clients.

Rivastigmine

(rye-va-**stig**-meen) Exelon, Exelon Patch

Classification: *Therapeutic:* Anti-Alzheimer's agents; *Pharmacological:* Cholinergics (cholinesterase inhibitors); *Pregnancy Category B*

Indications: *PO:* Mild to moderate dementia associated with Alzheimer's disease. *Transdermal:* Treatment of mild to moderate dementia associated with Alzheimer's and Parkinson's diseases.

Action: Enhances cholinergic function by reversible inhibition of cholinesterase. Does not cure the disease.

Pharmacokinetics: *Absorption:* Well absorbed following oral administration. Transdermal patch slowly absorbed over 8 hr. *Distribution:* Widely distributed. *Metabolism and Excretion:* Rapidly and extensively metabolized by liver; metabolites are excreted by kidneys.

T $\frac{1}{2}$: *PO:* 1.5 hr; *transdermal:* 24 hr.

TIME/ACTION PROFILE (improvement in dementia)

Route	Onset	Peak	Duration
PO	Within 2 wk	Up to 12 wk	Unknown
Transdermal	Unknown	Unknown	Unknown

Contraindicated in: Hypersensitivity to rivastigmine or other carbamates.

Use Cautiously in: History of asthma or obstructive pulmonary disease; history of GI bleeding; sick sinus syndrome or other supraventricular cardiac conduction abnormalities. *Transdermal:* Clients weighing <50 kg: at risk for ↑ adverse reactions; *Pregnancy/Lactation:* Safety not established.

Adverse Reactions/Side Effects: (CAPITALS) indicate life-threatening; underlines indicate most frequent).

CNS: Weakness, dizziness, drowsiness, headache, sedation (unusual). **CV:** Edema, heart failure, hypotension. **GI:** Anorexia, dyspepsia, nausea, vomiting, abdominal pain, diarrhea, flatulence, weight gain (unusual). **Neuro:** Tremor. **Misc:** Fever, weight loss.

Interactions: *Nicotine* use may ↑ metabolism and ↑ blood levels.

Dosage: PO (Adults): 1.5 mg twice daily initially; after at least 2 weeks, dose may be ↑ to 3 mg twice daily. Further increments may be made at 2-week intervals up to 6 mg twice daily. **Transdermal (Adults):** *Initial dose:* One patch 4.6 mg/24 hr initially. With good tolerability, after a minimum of 4 weeks, may ↑ to *maintenance dose* of one patch of 9.5 mg/24 hr.

Availability: Brand only

Capsules: 1.5 mg, 3 mg, 4.5 mg, 6 mg. **COST: $$$. Oral Solution:** 2 mg/mL in 120-mL bottle. **Transdermal Patch:** 4.6 mg/24 hr, 9.5 mg/24 hr.

● **Geriatric Considerations:** Be aware of GI side effects; may need to start with lower dose and titrate slowly.

● **Pediatric/Adolescent Considerations:** Safety not established. No indications.

● **Clinical Assessments:** Monitor for cognitive functions before and during treatment. Mini Mental State Examination (MMSE) and clock-drawing tests helpful screening tools.

> **Clinical Tips/Alerts:** Family members/caregivers with close contact better able to observe improvement/decline in cognition or behaviors. Always start *transdermal patch* at lowest dose, and titrate slowly. High doses associated with *significant GI reactions*, such as nausea, vomiting, diarrhea, anorexia/↓ appetite, and weight loss.

Selegiline Transdermal

(se-**le**-ji-leen) Emsam

Classification: *Therapeutic:* Antidepressants; *Pharmacological:* Monoamine oxidase type B inhibitors; *Pregnancy Category C*

Indications: Major depressive disorder.

Action: Following conversion by MAO to its active form, selegiline inactivates MAO by irreversibly binding to it at type B (brain) sites; results in higher levels of monoamine neurotransmitters in brain (dopamine, serotonin, norepinephrine).

Pharmacokinetics: *Absorption:* 25%–30% of patch content absorbed transdermally; blood levels higher than those following oral administration because less first-pass hepatic metabolism. *Distribution:* Rapidly distributes to all body tissues; crosses blood-brain barrier.

Metabolism and Excretion: Mostly metabolized by liver, primarily by CYP2A6, CYP2C9, and CYP3A4/5 enzyme systems; 10% excreted in urine as metabolites, 2% in feces; negligible renal excretion of unchanged drug.

$T^{1}/_{2}$: 18–25 hr.

TIME/ACTION PROFILE

Route	Onset	Peak	Duration
Transdermal	Unknown	2 or more wk	2 wk (after discontinuation)

Contraindicated in: Hypersensitivity; pheochromocytoma; concurrent SSRIs (fluoxetine, paroxetine, citalopram, escitalopram, and others), non-SSRIs (venlafaxine, duloxetine); tricyclic antidepressants (amitriptyline, imipramine, and others), carbamazepine, oxcarbazepine, amphetamines, vasoconstrictors (ephedrine, pseudoephedrine), bupropion, meperidine, tramadol, methadone, propoxyphene, dextromethorphan, mirtazapine cyclobenzaprine, other MAOIs (isocarboxazid, phenelzine, tranylcypromine), oral selegiline, sympathomimetic amines, amphetamines, cocaine or local anesthetics with vasoconstrictors; St. John's wort; alcohol.

DRUGS
R–Z

Use Cautiously in: Elective surgery within 10 days; benzodiazepines, mivacurium, rapacuronium, fentanyl, morphine and codeine may be used cautiously; history of mania; **dosing at 9 mg/24 hr or 12 mg/24 hr requires dietary modification** (avoid foods containing large amounts of tyramine); *Pregnancy:* Use only if benefit out-weighs risk to fetus. *Lactation:* Safety not established.

Adverse Reactions/Side Effects: (CAPITALS indicate life-threatening; underlines indicate most frequent.)

CNS: Insomnia, abnormal thinking, agitation, amnesia, worsening of mania/hypomania. **EENT:** Tinnitus. **Resp:** ↑ Cough. **CV:** HYPERTENSIVE CRISIS, chest pain, orthostatic hypotension, peripheral edema. **GI:** Diarrhea, altered taste, anorexia, constipation, flatulence, gastroenteritis, vomiting. **GU:** Dysmenorrhea, metrorrhagia, urinary frequency. **Derm:** Application site reactions, acne, ecchymoses, pruritus, sweating. **MS:** Myalgia, neck pain, pathological fracture. **Neuro:** Paresthesia.

Interactions: Concurrent SSRIs (fluoxetine, citalopram, escitalopram, and others), SNRIs (venlafaxine, duloxetine), tricyclic antidepressants (amitriptyline, imipramine, and others), carbamazepine, oxcarbazepine, amphetamines, vasocon-strictors (ephedrine, pseudoephedrine, phenylpropanolamine), bupropion, meperidine, tramadol, methadone, propoxyphene, dextromethorphan, mirtazapine, cyclobenzaprine, other MAOIs (isocarboxazid, phenelzine, tranylcypromine), oral selegiline, sympathomimetic amines, amphetamines, cocaine, or local anesthetics with vasoconstrictors; these may all ↑ risk of hypertensive crisis. **Drug-Natural:** St. John's wort may ↑ risk of hypertensive crisis.

Dosage: Transdermal (Adults): 6 mg/24 hr, if necessary, may be ↑ at intervals of 2 weeks, in increments of 3 mg, up to 12 mg/24 hr.

Availability: Brand only

Transdermal **Patch:** 6 mg/24 hr, 9 mg/24 hr, 12 mg/24 hr. COST: **$$$$**.

● **Geriatric Considerations:** Clients ≥65 yr may be more susceptible to orthostatic hypotension.

● **Pediatric/Adolescent Considerations:** Safety not established; may ↑ risk of suicide attempt/ideation esp. during early treatment or dose adjustment; risk may be greater in children or adolescents. Not approved for pediatric clients and should not be used in ages <12 yr.

● **Clinical Assessments:** Assess mental status and mood changes; monitor for suicidality early and during dosage adjustments. Monitor BP and pulse before and during treatment for significant changes.

Clinical Tips/Alerts: First transdermal patch for depression. Do not need to follow MAOI (tyramine-restricted) diet for doses of 6 mg/24 hr. *Need to follow MAOI diet with dosages of 9 mg/24 hr and 12 mg/24 hr to avoid hypertensive crisis (see MAOI diet in Tools tab). Hypertensive crisis signs and symptoms are:* chest pain, tachycardia or bradycardia, severe headache, neck stiffness or soreness, nausea and vomiting, sweating, photosensitivity, and enlarged pupils. Discontinue selegiline immediately, and (seek medical help) administer phentolamine 5 mg or labetalol 20 mg slowly IV to control hypertension. Do not use concurrently with other antidepressants (SSRIs, tricyclic antidepressants). Avoid using within 2 weeks of each other; 5 weeks after fluoxetine). (See *Serotonin Syndrome, Basics tab.*)

Sertraline

(**ser**-tra-leen) Zoloft

Classification: *Therapeutic:* antidepressants; *Pharmacological:* SSRIs; *Pregnancy Category C*

Indications: Major depressive disorder. Panic disorder. OCD, children 6–17 yr and adults. Post-traumatic stress disorder (PTSD). Social anxiety disorder (social phobia). PMDD. **Off-Label Use:** GAD.

Action: Inhibits neuronal uptake of serotonin in the CNS, thus potentiating activity of serotonin. Has little effect on norepinephrine or dopamine.

Pharmacokinetics: *Absorption:* Appears to be well absorbed after oral administration. *Distribution:* Extensively distributed throughout body tissues.

Metabolism and Excretion: Extensively metabolized by liver; one metabolite has some antidepressant activity; 14% excreted unchanged in feces.

Protein Binding: 98%.

T $\frac{1}{2}$: 24 hr.

TIME/ACTION PROFILE (antidepressant effect)

Route	Onset	Peak	Duration
PO	Within 2–4 wk	Unknown	Unknown

Contraindicated in: Hypersensitivity; concurrent MAOI therapy (may result in serious, potentially fatal, reactions); concurrent pimozide; oral concentrate contains alcohol and should be avoided in clients with known intolerance.

DRUGS
R-Z

Use Cautiously in: _Pregnancy and lactation:_ Severe hepatic or renal impairment; clients with a history of mania; clients at risk for suicide; children (↑ incidence of adverse CNS reactions).

Adverse Reactions/Side Effects: (CAPITALS indicate life-threatening; underlines indicate most frequent.)

CNS: Dizziness, drowsiness, fatigue, headache, insomnia, agitation, anxiety, confusion, emotional lability, impaired concentration, manic reaction, nervousness, weakness, yawning. **EENT :** Pharyngitis, rhinitis, tinnitus, visual abnormalities. **CV:** Chest pain, palpitations. **GI:** Diarrhea, dry mouth, nausea, abdominal pain, altered taste, anorexia, constipation, dyspepsia, flatulence, ↑ appetite, vomiting. **GU:** Sexual dysfunction, menstrual disorders, urinary disorders, urinary frequency. **Derm:** ↑ sweating, hot flashes, rash. **MS:** Back pain, myalgia. **Neuro:** Tremor, hypertonia, hypoesthesia, paresthesia, twitching. **Misc:** Fever, thirst.

Interactions: Potentially fatal reactions may occur with concurrent MAOIs. MAOIs should be stopped at least 14 days before sertraline therapy. Sertraline should be stopped at least 14 days before MAOI therapy. May ↑ pimozide levels and the risk of potentially life-threatening CV reactions. May ↑ sensitivity to adrenergics and ↑ risk of serotonin syndrome. Concurrent use with alcohol not recommended. May ↑ levels/effects of warfarin, phenytoin, tricyclic antidepressants, some benzodiazepines (alprazolam), clozapine, or tolbutamide. Cimetidine ↑ blood levels and effects. **Drug-Natural:** ↑ Risk of serotonergic side effects including serotonin syndrome with St. John's wort and SAMe.

Dosage: Depression/OCD: PO (Adults): 50 mg/day as a single dose in the morning or evening initially; after several weeks may be ↑ at weekly intervals up to 200 mg/day depending on response. **OCD: PO (Children 13–17 yr):** 50 mg once daily. May ↑ by 25–50 mg/day every week. Max: 200 mg/day. **OCD: PO (Children 6–12 yr):** 25 mg once daily, May ↑ by 25–50 mg/day every week. Max: 200 mg/day.

Panic Disorder: PO (Adults): 25 mg/day initially; may ↑ after 1 week to 50 mg/day.

PTSD: PO (Adults): 25 mg once daily for 7 days, then ↑ to 50 mg once daily; may be ↑ if needed at intervals of at least 7 days (range 50–200 mg once daily). **Social Anxiety Disorder: PO (Adults):** 25 mg once daily initially, then 50 mg once daily; may be ↑ at weekly intervals up to 200 mg/day.

PMDD: PO (Adults): 50 mg/day initially either daily or during luteal phase of cycle. Daily dosing may be titrated upward in 50-mg increments at the beginning of a cycle. In luteal phase—only dosing 50 mg/day on cycle days 15–28. Maximum: 100 mg/day. Note: Begin each cycle with 50 mg/day × 3 days.

Availability (generic available)

Tablets: 25 mg, 50 mg, 100 mg. COST: *Generic:* **$–$$. Capsules:** Canadian: 50 mg, 100 mg. **Oral concentrate (12% alcohol):** 20 mg/mL in 60–mL bottle. COST: **$–$$.**

- **Geriatric Considerations:** Some elderly may have greater sensitivity to adverse events; caution initially with dizziness/drowsiness; clinically significant hyponatremia possible.
- **Pediatric/Adolescent Considerations**: Not approved for children (except for OCD); benefit needs to outweigh risks. Monitor face to face for suicidality early and during dosage adjustments; ↑ risk for suicidality. Monitor for ↑ agitation and hyperexcitability. Do not stop abruptly; taper slowly to discontinue.
- **Clinical Assessments:** Monitor for changes in mood, for suicidality. Monitor changes using a depression rating scale before and after treatment. Diagnosis-based observations: OCD: reduction in compulsive behaviors/obsessive thoughts, etc.

Clinical Tips/Alerts: Potentially fatal reactions may occur with concurrent MAOIs. MAOIs should be stopped at least 14 days before sertraline therapy. Sertraline should be stopped at least 14 days before MAOI therapy (*see Serotonin Syndrome, Basics tab*). Antidepressants are also used for comorbid anxiety treatment.

Temazepam

(tem-**az**-a-pam) Restoril

Classification: *Therapeutic:* sedatives/hypnotics; *Pharmacological:* benzodiazepines; *Schedule IV; Pregnancy Category X*

Indications: Short-term management of insomnia (<4 wk).

Action: Acts at many levels in CNS, producing generalized depression. Effects may be mediated by GABA, an inhibitory neurotransmitter.

Pharmacokinetics: *Absorption:* Well absorbed after oral administration. *Distribution:* Widely distributed; crosses blood-brain barrier. Probably crosses placenta and enters breast milk. Accumulation of drug occurs with chronic dosing. *Metabolism and Excretion:* Metabolized by liver.

Protein Binding: 96%.

T $^1/_2$: 10–20 hr.

DRUGS R-Z

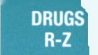

TIME/ACTION PROFILE (sedation)

Route	Onset	Peak	Duration
PO	30 min	2–3 hr	6–8 hr

Contraindicated in: Hypersensitivity; cross-sensitivity with other benzodiazepines may exist; pre-existing CNS depression; severe uncontrolled pain; angle-closure glaucoma; impaired respiratory function; sleep apnea. *Pregnancy:* Not safe during pregnancy; ↑ risk of birth defects in early pregnancy. Neonates born to mothers taking temazepam may experience withdrawal effects. *Lactation:* Infants may become sedated. Discontinue drug or bottle-feed.

Use Cautiously in: Pre-existing hepatic dysfunction; history of suicide attempt or drug addiction.

Adverse Reactions/Side Effects: (CAPITALS indicate life-threatening; <u>underlines</u> indicate most frequent.)

CNS: Abnormal thinking, behavior changes, <u>hangover</u>, dizziness, drowsiness, hallucinations, lethargy, paradoxic excitation, sleep—driving. **EENT:** Blurred vision. **GI:** Constipation, diarrhea, nausea, vomiting. **Derm:** Rashes. **Misc:** Physical dependence, psychological dependence, tolerance, ANAPHYLACTIC REACTION.

Interactions: ↑ CNS depression with *alcohol, antidepressants, antihistamines, opioid analgesics,* and other *sedatives/hypnotics.* May ↓ efficacy of *levodopa. Rifampin* or *smoking* ↑ metabolism and may ↓ effectiveness of temazepam. *Probenecid* may prolong effects of temazepam. Sedative effects may be ↓ by *theophylline.* **Drug-Natural:** Concomitant use of *kava, valerian, skullcap, chamomile,* or *hops* can ↑ CNS depression.

Dosage: PO (Adults): 15–30 mg at bedtime initially if needed; some clients may require only 7.5 mg.

PO (Geriatric or Debilitated Clients): 7.5 mg at bedtime.

Availability (generic available)

Capsules: 7.5 mg, 15 mg, 22.5 mg, 30 mg. COST: Generic **$**.

● **Geriatric Considerations:** Elderly clients have ↑ sensitivity to benzodiazepines. Appears on Beers list and associated with ↑ risk of falls (↓ dose required [7.5 mg at bedtime]).

● **Pediatric/Adolescent Considerations:** Safety and efficacy not established.

● **Substance Abuse Considerations:** Prolonged high-dose prescription may lead to psychological/physical dependence.

Temazepam

● **Clinical Assessments:** Assess sleep patterns before and during treatment.

> **Clinical Tips/Alerts:** Clients have been known to perform activities (cook/eat/drive) *while asleep* (complex sleep-related behaviors) and *serious allergic reactions* have happened (swelling of tongue/throat, difficulty breathing) requiring emergency care. If angioedema develops, seek emergency treatment and do not use drug again. Helpful for sleep-onset difficulty and night-time awakenings. Sleep disturbances can be manifestation of physical or psychiatric disorder; clients with insomnia that does not remit after 7–10 days of therapy should be evaluated for physical/psychiatric disorder; also if there is worsening of insomnia or behavioral abnormalities or new thinking.

Thiamine

(**thye**-a-min) Biamine, vitamin B$_1$, *Betaxin, Bewon*

Classification: *Therapeutic:* Vitamins; *Pharmacological:* Water-soluble vitamins; *Pregnancy Category A*

Indications: Treatment of thiamine deficiencies (beriberi). Prevention of Wernicke's encephalopathy. Dietary supplement for clients with GI disease, alcoholism, or cirrhosis.

Action: Required for carbohydrate metabolism.

Pharmacokinetics: *Absorption:* Well absorbed from GI tract by an active process. Excessive amounts not absorbed completely. Also well absorbed from IM sites.

Distribution: Widely distributed. Enters breast milk.

Metabolism and Excretion: Metabolized by liver. Excess amounts excreted unchanged by kidneys.

T $\frac{1}{2}$: Unknown.

TIME/ACTION PROFILE (time for symptoms of deficiency—edema and heart failure—to resolve*)

Route	Onset	Peak	Duration
PO, IM, IV	Hour	Days	Days–weeks

*Confusion and psychosis take longer to respond

Contraindicated in: Hypersensitivity; known alcohol intolerance or bisulfite hypersensitivity (elixir only).

DRUGS R-Z

DRUGS R-Z

Use Cautiously in: Wernicke's encephalopathy (condition may be worsened unless thiamine administered before glucose).

Adverse reactions and side effects are extremely rare and are usually associated with IV administration or extremely large doses.

CNS: Restlessness, weakness. **EENT:** Tightness of the throat. **Resp:** Pulmonary edema, respiratory distress. **CV:** VASCULAR COLLAPSE, hypotension, vasodilation. **GI:** GI bleeding, nausea. **Derm:** Cyanosis, pruritus, sweating, tingling, urticaria, warmth. **Misc:** ANGIOEDEMA.

Interactions: None significant.

Dosage: Thiamine Deficiency (Beriberi): PO (Adults): 5–10 mg three daily. **PO (Children):** 10–50 mg/day in divided doses. **IM, IV (Adults):** 5–100 mg three times daily. **IM, IV (Children):** 10–25 mg/day. **Dietary Supplement: PO (Adults):** 1–1.6 mg/day. **PO (Children 4–10 yr):** 0.9–1 mg/day. **PO (Children birth–3 yr):** 0.3–0.7 mg/day.

Availability (generic available)
Tablets: 5 mg OTC, 10 mg OTC, 25 mg OTC, 50 mg OTC, 100 mg OTC, 250 mg OTC, 500 mg OTC. COST: S. **Elixir** Canadian: 250 mcg/5 mL OTC. **Injection:** 100 mg/mL in 1-mL ampules and prefilled syringes and 1-, 2-, 10-, and 30-mL vials. ***In Combination With:*** Other vitamins, minerals, and trace elements in multivitamin preparations OTC.

● **Geriatric Considerations:** Evaluate alcohol intake and daily food intake.
● **Pediatric/Adolescent Considerations:** Thiamine deficiency develops if thiamine missing from diet. Need whole grain/enriched cereals and breads, fresh vegetables, and meat (esp. pork).
● **Clinical Assessments:** Assess client for signs and symptoms of thiamine deficiency (anorexia, GI distress, irritability, palpitations, tachycardia, edema, paresthesia, muscle weakness and pain, depression, memory loss, confusion, psychosis, visual disturbances, elevated serum pyruvic acid levels).

Clinical Tips/Alerts: Thiamine deficiency from malnutrition can develop in long-term alcoholics. Wernicke's encephalopathy caused by thiamine (vitamin B_1) deficiency. Classic triad is *encephalopathy, ataxic gait,* and *oculomotor dysfunction.* Wernicke's encephalopathy also associated with Korsakoff's psychosis and with potentially irreversible anterograde and retrograde amnesia. Parenteral thiamine may be needed until normal nutritional diet consistently followed.

Thioridazine

(thye-oh-**rid**-a-zeen) Mellaril, Mellaril-S, *Apo-Thioridazine, Novo-Ridazine, PMS Thioridazine*

Classification: *Therapeutic:* Antipsychotics; *Pharmacological:* Phenothiazines; *Pregnancy Category C*

Indications: Treatment of refractory schizophrenia. Considered second-line treatment after failure with atypical antipsychotics.

Action: Alters effects of dopamine in CNS. Possesses significant anticholinergic and alpha-adrenergic blocking activity.

Pharmacokinetics: *Absorption:* Absorption from tablets variable; may be better with oral liquid formulations.

Distribution: Widely distributed, high concentrations in CNS. Crosses placenta and enters breast milk.

Metabolism and Excretion : Highly metabolized by liver and GI mucosa.

Protein Binding: ≥90%.

T $^1/_2$: 21–24 hr.

TIME/ACTION PROFILE (antipsychotic effects)

Route	Onset	Peak	Duration
PO	Unknown	Unknown	8–12 hr

Contraindicated in: Hypersensitivity; cross-sensitivity with other phenothiazines may exist; angle-closure glaucoma; bone marrow depression; severe liver or CV disease; known alcohol intolerance (concentrate only); concurrent fluvoxamine, propranolol, pindolol, fluoxetine, other agents known to inhibit CYP450 2D6 enzyme, or agents known to prolong QTc interval (risk of life-threatening arrrhythmias); hypokalemia (correct condition before use); QTc interval >450 msec.

Use Cautiously in: Debilitated clients; glaucoma; urinary retention; diabetes mellitus; clients with risk factors for electrolyte imbalance (dehydration, diuretic therapy); respiratory disease; prostatic hyperplasia; CNS tumors; epilepsy; intestinal obstruction. *Pregnancy:* Safety not established. *Lactation:* Safety not established. Recommend discontinue drug or bottle-feed.

Adverse Reactions/Side Effects: (CAPITALS indicate life-threatening; underlines indicate most frequent.)

DRUGS
R–Z

CNS: NMS, sedation, extrapyramidal reactions, tardive dyskinesia. **EENT:** Blurred vision, dry eyes, lens opacities, pigmentary retinopathy (high doses). **CV:** ARRHYTHMIAS, QTc PROLONGATION, hypotension, tachycardia. **GI:** Constipation, dry mouth, anorexia, drug-induced hepatitis, ileus, weight gain. **GU:** Urinary retention, priapism. **Derm:** Photosensitivity, pigment changes, rashes. **Endo:** Galactorrhea, amenorrhea. **Hemat:** AGRANULOCYTOSIS, leukopenia. **Metab:** Hyperthermia. **Misc:** Allergic reactions.

Interactions: Concurrent *fluvoxamine*, *propranolol*, *pindolol*, *fluoxetine*, other agents known to inhibit *CYP450 2D6* enzyme, *or agents known to prolong QTc interval* (risk of life-threatening arrhythmias). *Diuretics* ↑ risk of electrolyte imbalance and arrhythmias. Additive hypotension with other *antihypertensives*, *nitrates*, and acute ingestion of *alcohol*. Additive CNS depression with other *CNS depressants*, including *alcohol*, *antihistamines*, *opioid analgesics*, *sedative/hypnotics*, and *general anesthetics*. Additive anticholinergic effects with other *drugs possessing anticholinergic properties*, including *antihistamines*, *antidepressants*, *atropine*, *haloperidol*, other *phenothiazines*, and *disopyramide*. *Lithium* ↓ blood levels of thioridazine. Thioridazine may mask early signs of *lithium* toxicity and ↑ risk of extrapyramidal reactions. ↑ Risk of agranulocytosis with *antithyroid agents*. Concurrent use with *epinephrine* may result in severe hypotension and tachycardia. May ↓ effectiveness of *levodopa*.

Dosage: PO (Adults and Children >12 yr): 50–100 mg three times daily initially; may be gradually ↑ to maintenance dose of up to 800 mg/day. **PO (Children):** 0.5 mg/kg/day in divided doses initially; may be gradually ↑ to maintenance dose of up to 3 mg/kg/day.

Availability (generic available)

Tablets: 10 mg, 15 mg, 25 mg, 50 mg, 100 mg, 150 mg, 200 mg. **COST: $. Oral Suspension:** Canadian: 10 mg/5 mL, 25 mg/5 mL, 100 mg/5 mL. **Concentrated Oral Solution:** 30 mg/mL, 100 mg/mL.

- **Geriatric Considerations:** Geriatric clients may be at ↑ risk for extrapyramidal and CNS adverse effects. Appears on Beers list. ↑ Risk of mortality in elderly with dementia-related psychosis.

- **Pediatric/Adolescent Considerations:** Since Black Box Warning for proarrhythmic effects, use in children should be avoided.

- **Clinical Assessments:** ECG before and periodically during treatment (QT prolongation) and during dosage adjustment. Also, BP, pulse, respiration, CBC, LFTs, eye examinations. Monitor mental status, mood, behavior. Weight, BMI, waist measurement, FBS, and lipids. (See BMI/Metabolic Syndrome, Tools tab.) Monitor for EPS, TD, NMS. (See Psychotropic Adverse Effects, Basics tab.)

Clinical Tips/Alerts: Thioridazine prescribed only if other antipsychotics fail as benefits do not outweigh risks. Prolongs QTc interval (dose-related) and associated with torsade de pointes–type arrhythmias and sudden death. Mellaril has been discontinued worldwide because of these serious side effects, but generic thioridazine available. Agranulocytosis occurs 4–10 wk of therapy with recovery 1–2 wk after discontinuation. ↑ Mortality in elderly with dementia-related psychosis.

Thiothixene

(thye-oh-**thix**-een) Navane

Classification: *Therapeutic:* Antipsychotics (conventional); *Pharmacological:* Thioxanthenes; *Pregnancy Category C*

Indications: Schizophrenia. Considered second-line treatment after failure with atypical antipsychotics. **Off-Label Use:** Other psychotic disorders, bipolar disorder.

Action: Alters effect of dopamine in CNS.

Pharmacokinetics: *Absorption:* Well absorbed following oral administration. *Distribution:* Widely distributed; crosses placenta. *Metabolism and Excretion:* Mainly metabolized by liver.

T $^{1}/_{2}$: 30 hr.

TIME/ACTION PROFILE (antipsychotic effects)

Route	Onset	Peak	Duration
PO	Days-weeks	Unknown	Unknown
IM	1–6 hr	Unknown	Unknown

Contraindicated in: Hypersensitivity to thiothixene or other phenothiazines (cross-sensitivity may occur); circulatory collapse; blood dyscrasias; CNS depression.

Use Cautiously in: Geriatric or debilitated clients (initial dosage reduction may be required); diabetes mellitus; respiratory disease; prostatic hypertrophy; CNS tumors; epilepsy; intestinal obstruction. *Pregnancy:* Safety not established. *Lactation:* Safety not established. Discontinue drug or bottle-feed.

Adverse Reactions/Side Effects: (CAPITALS indicate life-threatening; underlines indicate most frequent.)

CNS: NMS, extrapyramidal reactions, sedation, tardive dyskinesia, seizures. **EENT:** Blurred vision, dry eyes, lens opacities. **CV:** Hypotension, tachycardia, nonspecific

DRUGS
R-Z

Clinical Tips/Alerts: This should not be a first-line treatment. ↑ Mortality in elderly with dementia-related psychosis.

Clinical Assessments: Monitor BP, pulse, respiration, CBCs (leukopenia), LFTs (hepatotoxicity), eye examinations. Monitor mental status, mood, behavior, positive/negative symptoms. Weight, BMI, waist measurement, FBS, and lipids. (See BMI/Metabolic Syndrome, *Tools tab*.) Monitor for EPS, TD, NMS. (See *Psychotropic Adverse Effects, Basics tab.*)

Pediatric/Adolescent Considerations: Safety not established. No indications for children.

● **Geriatric Considerations:** Consider initial dosage reduction. ↑ Risk for falls (sedation). ↑ Risk of mortality in elderly with dementia-related psychosis.

Availability (generic available)
Capsules: 1 mg, 2 mg, 5 mg, 10 mg, 20 mg. COST: **$**. **Concentrated Oral Solution:** 5 mg/mL in 30- and 120-mL containers.

Dosage: PO (Adults): *Mild conditions:* 2 mg three times daily (up to 15 mg/day if necessary); *severe conditions:* 5 mg twice daily (up to 20–30 mg/day; not to exceed 60 mg/day).

Drug-Natural: Concomitant use of kava, valerian, skullcap, chamomile, or hops can ↑ CNS depression. ↑ Risk of cardiac effects with quinidine. May ↑ effectiveness of levodopa. ↑ CNS depression.

Interactions: Additive hypotension with antihypertensives, acute ingestion of alcohol, and nitrates. Additive hypotension may occur if epinephrine is given to treat hypotension. Additive CNS depression with other CNS depressants, including alcohol, antihistamines, antidepressants, opioid analgesics, and sedatives/hypnotics. Additive anticholinergic effects with other drugs having anticholinergic properties, including antihistamines, antidepressants, quinidine, and disopyramide. May ↑ effectiveness of levodopa.

GI: Constipation, dry mouth, anorexia, ileus, nausea. **GU:** Urinary retention. **Derm:** Photosensitivity, pigment changes, rashes. **Endo:** Breast enlargement, galactorrhea. **Hemat:** Leukocytosis, leukopenia. **Metab:** Hyperpyrexia. **Misc:** Allergic reactions.

ECG changes.

Topiramate

(toe-**peer**-i-mate) Topamax

Classification: *Therapeutic:* anticonvulsants, mood stabilizers; *Pregnancy Category C*

Indications: Seizures including: partial-onset, primary generalized tonic-clonic, seizures due to Lennox-Gastaut syndrome. Prevention of migraine headache in adults. **Off-Label Use:** Adjunct in treatment of bipolar disorder.

Action: Action may be due to: Blockade of sodium channels in neurons; enhancement of GABA, an inhibitory neurotransmitter; prevention of activation of excitatory receptors.

Pharmacokinetics: *Absorption:* Well absorbed (80%) after oral administration. *Distribution:* Unknown.

Metabolism and Excretion: 70% excreted unchanged in urine.

T $^1/_2$: 21 hr.

TIME/ACTION PROFILE (blood levels*)

Route	Onset	Peak	Duration
PO	Unknown	2 hr	12 hr

*After single dose.

Contraindicated in: Hypersensitivity; *Lactation.*

Use Cautiously in: Renal impairment (dosage reduction recommended if CCr <70 mL/min/1.73 m²); hepatic impairment; dehydration; *Pregnancy:* Use at lower doses only if maternal benefit outweighs fetal risk; possible ↑ risk for congenital malformations (Meador 2006). *Lactation:* Discontinue drug or bottle-feed.

Adverse Reactions/Side Effects: (CAPITALS indicate life-threatening; underlines indicate most frequent.)

CNS: ↑ SEIZURES, dizziness, drowsiness, fatigue, impaired concentration/memory, nervousness, psychomotor slowing, speech problems, sedation, aggressive reaction, agitation, anxiety, cognitive disorders, confusion, depression, malaise, mood problems. **EENT:** Abnormal vision, diplopia, nystagmus, acute myopia/secondary angle-closure glaucoma. **GI:** Nausea, abdominal pain, anorexia, constipation, dry mouth. **GU:** Kidney stones. **Derm:** Oligohydrosis (↑ in children). **F and E:** Hyperchloremic metabolic acidosis. **Hemat:** Leukopenia. **Metab:** Weight loss, hyperthermia (↑ in children). **Neuro:** Ataxia, paresthesia, tremor. **Misc:** SUICIDE ATTEMPT, fever.

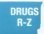

Interactions: Blood levels may be ↑ by *phenytoin, carbamazepine,* or *valproic acid.* May ↑ blood levels and effects of *phenytoin* or *amitriptyline.* May ↑ blood levels and effects of *hormonal contraceptives, risperidone, lithium,* or *valproic acid.* ↑ Risk of CNS depression with *alcohol* or other *CNS depressants.* Carbonic anhydrase inhibitors *(acetazolamide)* may ↑ risk of kidney stones. Concurrent use with *valproic acid* may ↑ risk of hyperammonemia/encephalopathy.

Dosage: **Epilepsy (monotherapy): PO (Adults and Children ≥10 yr):** *Seizures/ migraine prevention:* 50 mg/day initially, gradually ↑ over 6 wk to 400 mg/day in two divided doses. **Epilepsy (Adjunctive Therapy): PO (Adults and Children≥ 17 yr):** 25–50 mg/day ↑ by 25–50 mg/day at weekly intervals up to 200–400 mg/day in two divided doses (200–400 mg/day in two divided doses for partial seizures and 400 mg/day in two divided doses for primary generalized tonic/clonic seizures).

Renal Impairment: PO (Adults): *CCr <70 mL/min:* 50% of the usual dose.

PO (Children 2–17 yr): *Seizures:* 5–9 mg/kg/day in two divided doses; initiate with 25 mg (or less, based on 1–3 mg/kg) nightly for 7 days, then ↑ at intervals of 1–2 wk in increments of 1–3 mg/kg/day in two divided doses; titration should be based on clinical outcome.

Migraine Prevention: PO (Adults): 25 mg at night initially, ↑ by 25 mg/day at weekly intervals up to target dose of 100 mg/day in two divided doses.

Availability (generic available)
Sprinkle Capsules: 15 mg, 25 mg. COST: $$–$$$$. **Tablets:** 25 mg, 50 mg, 100 mg, 200 mg. COST: $$$$.

- **Geriatric Considerations:** Caution with drowsiness, confusion (falls); dosage reduction with renal impairment.
- **Pediatric/Adolescent Considerations:** Children are more prone to oligohydrosis and hyperthermia; safety in children <2 yr not established. No psychiatric use in children.
- **Clinical Assessments:** Assess mental status (mood); Young Mania Rating Scale (YMRS) before and during treatment. Monitor CBC with differential and platelets; may cause anemia. Monitor for suicidality.

> **Clinical Tips/Alerts:** Considered an adjunct to other mood stabilizers rather than effective as monotherapy for bipolar mania or depression. Helpful with weight loss.

Tranylcypromine

(tran-ill-**sip**-roe-meen) Parnate

Classification: *Therapeutic:* antidepressants; *Pharmacological:* MAOI; *Pregnancy Category C*

Indications: Treatment of major depressive episode without melancholia (usually reserved for clients who do not tolerate or respond to other modes of therapy [e.g., tricyclic antidepressants, SSRIs, SNRIs, or electroconvulsive therapy]).

Action: Inhibits enzyme monoamine oxidase, resulting in accumulation of various neurotransmitters (dopamine, epinephrine, norepinephrine, and serotonin).

Pharmacokinetics: *Absorption:* Unknown.

Distribution: Crosses placenta and enters breast milk.

T $^1/_2$: 90–190 min.

TIME/ACTION PROFILE (antidepressant effect)

Route	Onset	Peak	Duration
PO	2 days–3 wk	2–3 wk	3–5 days

Contraindicated in: Hypersensitivity; liver disease; cerebrovascular disease; CV disease; hypertension; pheochromocytoma; clients undergoing elective surgery requiring general anesthesia (should be discontinued at least 10 days before surgery); history of headache; excessive consumption of caffeine; concurrent use of meperidine, SSRI antidepressants, SNRI antidepressants, tricyclic antidepressants, tetracyclic antidepressants, nefazodone, trazodone, procarbazine, selegiline, linezolid, carbamazepine, cyclobenzaprine, bupropion, buspirone, sympathomimetics, other MAOIs, dextromethorphan, narcotics, alcohol, general anesthetics, diuretics, antihistamines, or tryptophan; concurrent use of foods containing high concentrations of tyramine; *lactation.*

Use Cautiously in: Clients who may be suicidal or have a history of drug dependency; hyperthyroidism; schizophrenia; bipolar disorder; seizure disorders; renal dysfunction; diabetes (↑ risk of hypoglycemia). *Pregnancy:* Safety not established.

Adverse Reactions/Side Effects: (CAPITALS indicate life-threatening; underlines indicate most frequent.)

CNS: SEIZURES, confusion, dizziness, drowsiness, headache, insomnia, restlessness, tremor, paresthesia, weakness. **EENT:** Blurred vision, tinnitus. **CV:** HYPERTENSIVE

DRUGS R-Z

CRISIS, edema, orthostatic hypotension, tachycardia. **GI:** Abdominal pain, anorexia, constipation, diarrhea, dry mouth, hepatitis, nausea. **GU:** Sexual dysfunction, urinary retention. **Hemat:** AGRANULOCYTOSIS, leukopenia, thrombocytopenia. **Derm:** Alopecia, rashes. **MS:** Muscle spasm.

Interactions: Potentially fatal adverse reactions may occur with concurrent use of other antidepressants, carbamazepine, cyclobenzaprine, sibutramine, procarbazine, or selegiline. Avoid using within 2 wk of each other (wait 5 wk from end of fluoxetine therapy). Hypertensive crisis may occur with amphetamines, methyldopa, levodopa, dopamine, epinephrine, norepinephrine, reserpine, methylphenidate, or vasoconstrictors. Hypertension or hypotension, coma, seizures, respiratory depression, and death may occur with meperidine (avoid using within 2–3 wk of MAOI therapy). Concurrent use with dextromethorphan may produce psychosis or bizarre behavior. Hypertension may occur with concurrent use of buspirone; avoid using within 2 wk of each other. Additive hypotension may occur with antihypertensives, spinal anesthesia, opioids, or barbiturates. Additive hypoglycemia may occur with insulins or oral hypoglycemic agents. Risk of seizures may be ↑ with tramadol. Serious, potentially fatal adverse effects (serotonin syndrome) may occur with concomitant use of St. John's wort and SAMe. Hypertensive crises may occur with large amounts of caffeine-containing herbs (cola nut, guarana, or malt) Insomnia, headache, tremor, hypomania may occur with ginseng. Hypertensive crises, disorientation, and memory impairment may occur with tryptophan or supplements containing tyrosine or phenylalanine. **Drug-Food:** Hypertensive crisis may occur with ingestion of foods containing high concentrations of tyramine (see Tools tab). Consumption of foods or beverages with high caffeine content ↑ risk of hypertension and arrhythmias.

Dosage: PO (Adults): 30 mg/day in two divided doses (morning and afternoon); after 2 wk can ↑ by 10 mg/day, at intervals of 1–3 wk, up to 60 mg/day.

Availability (generic available)
Tablets: 10 mg. COST: $$

● **Geriatric Considerations:** Elderly have greater sensitivity to adverse effects; evaluate for ability to follow diet.
● **Pediatric/Adolescent Considerations:** Safety and effectiveness not established. Monitor face for suicidality early in treatment and during dosage adjustments. No indications for use in children.
● **Clinical Assessments:** Assess/monitor for mood improvement, suicidality; monitor BP and pulse before and during treatment, weight, waist circumference, and BMI

before and during prescription. Other tests: FBS, lipids. (See *BMI/Metabolic Syndrome, Tools tab.*)

> **Clinical Tips/Alerts:** Potentially fatal reactions (serotonin syndrome) with concurrent use of other *antidepressants (SSRIs, SNRIs, bupropion, tricyclics, tetracyclics, nefazodone, trazodone), carbamazepine, cyclobenzaprine, sibutramine, linezolid, procarbazine,* or *selegiline.* Avoid using within at least 2 wk of each other (wait 5 wk from end of *fluoxetine* therapy). (*See serotonin syndrome, Basics tab.*) Client **must be willing to follow MAOI (tyramine-restricted) diet** to avoid hypertensive crisis [*emergency*]. (See MAOI diet, *Tools tab.*) Avoid *meperidine.* Although not a first-line treatment, should be considered for treatment-resistant depression. Associated with weight gain and sedation.

Trazodone

(**traz**-oh-done) Desyrel, Trialodine, Trazon

Classification : *Therapeutic:* Antidepressants; *Pregnancy Category C*

Indications: Major depression (children and adults). **Off-Label Use:** Insomnia; chronic pain syndromes, including diabetic neuropathy, and anxiety.

Action: Alters effects of serotonin in CNS.

Pharmacokinetics: *Absorption:* Well absorbed after oral administration. *Distribution:* Widely distributed.

Metabolism and Excretion: Extensively metabolized by liver (CYP3A4 enzyme system); minimal excretion of unchanged drug by kidneys.

Protein Binding: 89%–95%.

T $^1/_2$: 5–9 hr.

TIME/ACTION PROFILE (antidepressant effect)

Route	Onset	Peak	Duration
PO	1–2 wk	2–4 wk	Weeks

Contraindicated in: Hypersensitivity; recovery period after MI; concurrent electroconvulsive therapy.

Use Cautiously in: CV disease; suicidal behavior; may ↑ risk of suicide attempt/ideation esp. during early treatment or dose adjustment; severe hepatic or renal disease (dose reduction recommended); *Lactation:* Discontinue drug or bottle-feed.

DRUGS
R-Z

DRUGS R-Z

Adverse Reactions/Side Effects: (CAPITALS indicate life-threatening; underlines indicate most frequent.) <u>CNS</u>: Drowsiness, confusion, dizziness, fatigue, hallucinations, headache, insomnia, nightmares, slurred speech, syncope, weakness. **EENT:** Blurred vision, tinnitus. **CV:** Hypotension, arrhythmias, chest pain, hypertension, palpitations, tachycardia. **GI:** Dry mouth, altered taste, constipation, diarrhea, excess salivation, flatulence, nausea, vomiting. **GU:** Hematuria, erectile dysfunction, priapism, urinary frequency. **Derm:** Rashes. **Hemat:** Anemia, leukopenia. **MS:** Myalgia. **Neuro:** Tremor.

Interactions: May ↑ *digoxin* or *phenytoin* serum levels. ↑ CNS depression with other *CNS depressants*, including *alcohol*, *opioid analgesics*, and *sedatives/hypnotics*. ↑ Hypotension with *antihypertensives*, acute ingestion of *alcohol*, or *nitrates*. Concurrent use with *fluoxetine* ↑ levels and risk of toxicity from trazodone. Drugs that inhibit *CYP3A4 enzyme system*, including *ritonavir*, *indinavir*, and *ketoconazole*, ↑ levels and risk of toxicity. Drugs that induce *CYP3A4 enzyme system*, including *carbamazepine*, ↑ levels and may ↓ effectiveness. Do not use within 14 days of *MAOI* therapy. May ↑ prothrombin time with *warfarin*. **Drug-Natural:** Concomitant use of *kava*, *valerian*, or *chamomile* can ↑ CNS depression. ↑ Risk of serotonergic side effects, including serotonin syndrome, with *St. John's wort* and *SAMe*.

Dosage: PO (Adults): *Depression:* 150 mg/day in three divided doses; ↑ by 50 mg/day every 3–4 days until desired response (not to exceed 400 mg/day in outpatients or 600 mg/day in hospitalized clients). **PO (Children 12–18 yr):** *Depression:* 25 mg two to three time daily. Max: 400 mg/day. *Insomnia:* 25–100 mg/day at bedtime. **PO (Geriatric Clients):** 75 mg/day in divided doses initially; may be ↑ every 3–4 days.

Availability (generic available)
Tablets: 50 mg, 100 mg, 150 mg, 300 mg. COST: **$.**

● **Geriatric Considerations:** Initial dose reduction; drowsiness, hypotension may result in falls.

● **Pediatric/Adolescent Considerations:** Monitor face to face for suicidality early in treatment and during dosage adjustments; ↑ risk for suicidality. Rarely used to treat depression in children; may be used at lower doses for treatment of insomnia.

● **Clinical Assessments:** Assess/monitor for mood improvement, suicidality; monitor BP and pulse before and during *treatment*, baseline ECG and then periodically with pre-existing CV disease.

[**Clinical Tips/Alerts:** Trazodone often used for insomnia; concurrent use with *fluoxetine* can result in toxicity; do not use within 14 days of *MAOIs. Priapism* (sustained erection for hours) is an emergency and requires immediate medical treatment. Monitor for clinical worsening; unusual behaviors and suicidality.]

Triazolam

(trye-**az**-oh-lam) Halcion, *Apo-Triazo, Gen-Triazolam, Novo-Triolam, Nu-Triazo*

Classification: *Therapeutic:* Sedatives/hypnotics; *Pharmacological:* Benzodiazepines; *Schedule IV; Pregnancy Category X*

Indications: Short-term management of insomnia.

Action: Acts at many levels in CNS, producing generalized depression. Effects may be mediated by GABA, an inhibitory neurotransmitter.

Pharmacokinetics: *Absorption:* Well absorbed following oral administration. *Distribution:* Widely distributed; crosses blood-brain barrier. Probably crosses placenta and enters breast milk.

Metabolism and Excretion: Metabolized by liver.

Protein Binding: 89%.

T $^1/_2$: 1.6–5.4 hr.

TIME/ACTION PROFILE (sedation)

Route	Onset	Peak	Duration
PO	15–30 min	6–8 hr	Unknown

Contraindicated in: *Pregnancy, lactation, and children;* hypersensitivity; cross-sensitivity with other benzodiazepines may occur; pre-existing CNS depression; uncontrolled severe pain. **Use Cautiously in:** Pre-existing hepatic dysfunction (dose reduction recommended); history of suicide attempt or drug addiction.

Adverse Reactions/Side Effects: (CAPITALS indicate life-threatening; underlines indicate most frequent.)

CNS: Abnormal thinking, behavior changes, dizziness, excessive sedation, hangover, headache, anterograde amnesia, confusion, hallucinations, sleep-driving, lethargy, mental depression, paradoxical excitation. **EENT:** Blurred vision. **GI:** Constipation, diarrhea, nausea, vomiting. **Derm:** Rashes. **Misc:** Physical dependence, psychological dependence, tolerance.

Trihexyphenidyl

(trye-hex-ee-**fen**-i-dill) Artane, Trihexane, Trihexy, Apo-Trihex, PMS-Trihexyphenidyl.

Classification: *Therapeutic:* Antiparkinsonian agents; *Pharmacological:* Anticholinergics.

Pregnancy Category C

Interactions: Cimetidine, erythromycin, fluconazole, itraconazole, ketoconazole, indinavir, nelfinavir, ritonavir, or saquinavir may ↑ metabolism and enhance actions of triazolam; combination should be avoided. Additive CNS depression with *alcohol,* *antidepressants, antihistamines,* and *opioid analgesics.* May ↑ effectiveness of *levodopa.* May ↑ toxicity of *zidovudine. Isoniazid* may ↑ excretion and ↑ effects of triazolam. Sedative effects may be ↑ by *theophylline.*

Drug-Natural: Concomitant use of *kava, valerian, chamomile,* or *hops* can ↓ CNS depression. *Grapefruit juice* significantly ↑ blood levels and effects.

Drug-Food: *Grapefruit juice* significantly ↑ blood levels and effects.

Dosage: PO (Adults): 125–250 mcg (up to 500 mcg) at bedtime.

PO (Geriatric or Debilitated Clients): 125 mcg at bedtime initially; may be ↑ as needed.

Availability (generic available)

Tablets: 125 mcg, 250 mcg. COST: $.

- **Geriatric Considerations:** Elderly clients have ↓ sensitivity to benzodiazepines. Appears on Beers list and associated with ↑ risk of falls ↑ dose required [7.5 mg at bedtime]).

- **Pediatric/Adolescent Considerations:** Safety and efficacy not established. Not used in children.

- **Substance Abuse Considerations:** Prolonged high-dose treatment may lead to psychological/physical dependence.

- **Clinical Assessments:** Assess sleep patterns before and during treatment.

- **Clinical Tips/Alerts:** Clients have been known to perform activities (cook/eat/drive) *while asleep* (complex sleep-related behaviors) and *serious allergic reactions* have happened (swelling of tongue/throat, difficulty breathing) requiring emergency care. If angioedema develops, seek emergency treatment and do not use drug again. Helpful for sleep-onset difficulty and nighttime awakenings. Sleep disturbances can be manifestation of a physical or psychiatric disorder; clients with insomnia that does not remit after 7–10 days of therapy should be evaluated for physical/psychiatric disorder; also if worsening of insomnia or behavioral abnormalities or new thinking.

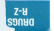

Indications: Adjunct in management of Parkinson syndrome of many causes, including drug-induced parkinsonism; drug-induced extrapyramidal effects.

Action: Inhibits action of acetylcholine, resulting in ↓ sweating and salivation, mydriasis (pupillary dilation), ↑ heart rate. Also has spasmolytic action on smooth muscle. Inhibits cerebral motor centers and blocks efferent impulses.

Pharmacokinetics: *Absorption:* Well absorbed following oral administration. *Distribution:* Unknown.
Metabolism and Excretion: Excreted mostly in urine.
T $\frac{1}{2}$: 3.7 hr.

TIME/ACTION PROFILE (anti-Parkinson effects)

Route	Onset	Peak	Duration
PO	1 hr	2–3 hr	6–12 hr
PO-ER	Unknown	Unknown	12–24 hr

Contraindicated in: Hypersensitivity; angle-closure glaucoma; acute hemorrhage; tachycardia secondary to cardiac insufficiency; thyrotoxicosis; known alcohol intolerance (elixir only).

Use Cautiously in: Geriatric and very young clients (↑ risk of adverse reactions); intestinal obstruction or infection; prostatic hyperplasia; chronic renal, hepatic, pulmonary, or cardiac disease. *Pregnancy, lactation, and children (safety not established).*

Adverse Reactions/Side Effects: (CAPITALS indicate life-threatening; underlines indicate most frequent.)

CNS: Dizziness, nervousness, confusion, drowsiness, headache, psychoses, weakness. **EENT:** Blurred vision, mydriasis. **CV:** Orthostatic hypotension, tachycardia. **GI:** Dry mouth, nausea, constipation, vomiting. **GU:** Urinary hesitancy, urinary retention. **Derm:** ↓ Sweating.

Interactions: Additive anticholinergic effects with *drugs having anticholinergic properties,* including *phenothiazines, tricyclic antidepressants, quinidine,* and *disopyramide.* May ↑ efficacy of *levodopa* but may ↑ risk of psychoses. Additive CNS depression with *CNS depressants,* including *alcohol, antihistamines, opioids,* and *sedatives/hypnotics.* Anticholinergics may alter absorption of other *orally administered drugs* by slowing motility of GI tract. *Antacids* may ↓ absorption. May ↑ GI mucosal lesions in clients taking *solid oral potassium chloride preparations.*

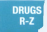

DRUGS R–Z

Drug-Natural: ↑ anticholinergic effects with *angel's trumpet, jimson weed,* and *scopolia.*

Dosage: PO (Adults): 1–2 mg/day initially; ↑ by 2 mg every 3–5 days. Usual maintenance dose 6–10 mg/day in three divided doses (up to 15 mg/day). Extended-release (Artane Sequels) preparations may be given every 12 hr after daily dose has been determined using conventional tablets or liquid.

Availability (generic available)

Tablets: 2 mg, 5 mg. COST: **$.** **Elixir (lime-mint flavor):** 2 mg/5 mL. **Extended-Release Capsules:** 5 mg.

- **Geriatric Considerations:** ↑ Risk of adverse effects; sensitive to anticholinergic effects. Caution with BPH (urinary retention); Risk for falls (dizziness, drowsiness).
- **Pediatric/Adolescent Considerations:** Safety not established. Not used in children.
- **Substance Abuse Considerations:** With alcohol, opioid, sedative use/ dependence, ↑ risk of adverse events. ↑ Risk for falls, dizziness, fatigue.
- **Clinical Assessments:** Assess for EPS before and during prescription. Monitor for improvement of symptoms (tremors, rigidity). (See *Psychotropic Adverse Effects, Basics tab.*)

Clinical Tips/Alerts: Do not use extended-release capsules until maintenance established with immediate-release tablets. *Taper gradually* when discontinuing to avoid *withdrawal* (anxiety, tachycardia, insomnia, return of Parkinson or extrapyramidal symptoms).

Valproates

divalproex sodium (dye-val-**proe**-ex **soe**-dee-um) Depakote ER, *Apo-Divalproex, DOM-Divalproex, Epival, Gen-Divalproex, Novo-Divalproex, Nu-Divalproex, PHL-Divalproex, PMS-Divalproex*

valproate sodium (val-**proe**-ate **soe**-dee-um) Depacon

valproic acid (val-**proe**-ik **as**-id) Depakene, *Apo-Valproic, DOM-Valproic Acid, PHL-Valproic Acid, PMS-Valproic Acid, Ratio-Valprox*

Classification: Therapeutic: Anticonvulsants; vascular headache suppressants; *Pregnancy Category D*

Indications: Monotherapy and adjunctive therapy for simple and complex absence seizures. Monotherapy and adjunctive therapy for complex partial seizures. Adjunctive therapy for clients with multiple seizure types, including absence seizures.

Divalproex sodium only: Manic episodes associated with bipolar disorder; prevention of migraine headache.

Action: ↑ Levels of GABA, inhibitory neurotransmitter in CNS.

Pharmacokinetics: *Absorption:* Well absorbed following oral administration; divalproex enteric-coated, and absorption delayed. ER form produces lower blood levels. IV administration results in complete bioavailability.

Distribution: Rapidly distributed into plasma and extracellular water. Crosses blood-brain barrier and placenta; enters breast milk.

Metabolism and Excretion : Mostly metabolized by liver; minimal amounts excreted unchanged in urine. **Protein binding:** 80%–90%; ↓ in neonates, elderly, renal impairment, or chronic hepatic disease.

$T^{1}/_{2}$: Adults: 9–16 hr.

TIME/ACTION PROFILE (onset = anticonvulsant effect; peak = blood levels)

Route	Onset	Peak	Duration
PO: Liquid	2–4 days	15–120 min	6–24 hr
PO: Capsules	2–4 days	1–4 hr	6–24 hr
PO: Delayed-release products	2–4 days	3–5 hr	12–24 hr
PO: Extended-release products	2–4 days	7–14 hr	24 hr
IV	2–4 days	End of infusion	6–24 hr

Contraindicated in: Hypersensitivity; hepatic impairment; known/suspected urea cycle disorders (may result in fatal hyperammonemic encephalopathy).

Use Cautiously in: Bleeding disorders; history of liver disease; organic brain disease; bone marrow depression; renal impairment. *Pregnancy:* Use during pregnancy linked to congenital anomalies, neural tube defects, clotting abnormalities, and hepatic dysfunction in the neonate. Should not be first-choice drug, linked to lower IQ (Meador, 2009). *Lactation:* Valproates pass into breast milk. Consider discontinuing nursing when valproates administered to nursing mother.

Adverse Reactions/Side Effects: (CAPITALS indicate life-threatening; underlines indicate most frequent.)

CNS: <u>Agitation</u>, <u>dizziness</u>, <u>headache</u>, <u>insomnia</u>, <u>sedation</u>, confusion, depression. **CV:** Peripheral edema. **EENT:** <u>Visual disturbances</u>. **GI:** HEPATOTOXICITY, PANCREATITIS, <u>abdominal pain</u>, <u>anorexia</u>, <u>diarrhea</u>, <u>indigestion</u>, <u>nausea</u>, <u>vomiting</u>, constipation,

DRUGS
R–Z

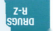

↑ appetite. **Derm:** Alopecia, rashes. **Endo:** Weight gain. **Hemat:** Leukopenia, throm-bocytopenia. **Metab:** HYPERAMMONEMIA. **Neuro:** Tremor, ataxia.

Interactions: ↑ Risk of bleeding with *warfarin*. Blood levels and toxicity may be ↓ by *aspirin, carbamazepine, chlorpromazine, cimetidine, erythromycin,* or *felbamate*. ↑ CNS depression with other *CNS depressants,* including *alcohol, antihistamines, anti-depressants, opioid analgesics, MAO inhibitors,* and *sedatives/hypnotics*. *MAOIs* and other *antidepressants* may ↑ seizure threshold and ↓ effectiveness of valproate. *Carbamazepine, meropenem, phenobarbital, phenytoin,* and *rifampin* may ↓ val-proate blood levels. Valproate may ↑ toxicity of *carbamazepine, diazepam, amitripty-line, nortriptyline, ethosuximide, lamotrigine, phenobarbital, phenytoin, topiramate,* and *zidovudine*.

Dosage: Regular-release and delayed-release formulations usually given in two to four divided doses daily; extended-release formulation (Depakote ER) usually given once daily.

Mood Stabilizer: PO (Adults): *Depakote:* Initial dose 750 mg/day in divided doses, titrated rapidly to desired clinical effect or trough plasma levels of 50–125 mcg/mL. *Depakote ER:* Initial dose 25 mg/kg once daily, titrated rapidly to desired clinical effect of trough plasma lev-els of 85–125 mcg/mL; [plasma level for mania] (dose not to exceed 60 mg/kg/day).

Anticonvulsant: PO (Adults and Children >10 yr): *Single-agent therapy* (complex partial seizures): Initial dose 10–15 mg/kg/day in one to four divided doses; ↑ by 5–10 mg/kg/day weekly until therapeutic response achieved (not to exceed 60 mg/kg/day); when daily dosage exceeds 250 mg, give in divided doses. *Polytherapy* (complex partial seizures): Initial dose 10–15 mg/kg/day; ↑ by 5–10 mg/kg/day weekly until therapeutic response achieved (not to exceed 60 mg/kg/day); when daily dosage exceeds 250 mg, give in divided doses.

PO (Adults and Children >2 yr [>10 yr for Depakote ER]): *Simple and complex absence seizures:* Initial dose 15 mg/kg/day in one to four divided doses; ↑ by 5–10 mg/kg/day weekly until therapeutic response achieved (not to exceed 60 mg/kg/day); when daily dosage exceeds 250 mg, give in divided doses.

Availability (generic available)
Valproic Acid (generic available)
Capsules: 250 mg, Canadian: 500 mg. COST: *Generic $.* **Syrup:** 250 mg/5 mL. COST: *Generic $.*

Valproate Sodium
Injection: 100 mg/mL in 5-mL vials.
Divalproex Sodium
Delayed-Release Tablets (Depakote): 125 mg, 250 mg, 500 mg. COST: **$$–$$$$**.
Capsules-sprinkle: 125 mg. COST: **$$. Extended-Release Tablets (Depakote ER):** 250 mg, 500 mg. COST: **$$–$$$.**

- **Geriatric Considerations:** ↑ Risk of adverse effects; dizziness, sedation (risk for falls). Do not use with hepatic impairment.
- **Pediatric/Adolescent Considerations:** Use cautiously in children, esp. <2 yr (at ↑ risk for potentially fatal hepatotoxicity). Psychiatric use in children based on safety profile for pediatric epilepsy. Monitor closely. Therapeutic range for pediatric mood stablization: Serum level 50–100 mcg/mL.
- **Clinical Assessments:** Assess mental status, mood; assess for suicidality. Monitor hepatic function (LDH, aspartate aminotransferase, alanine aminotransferase, and bilirubin) and serum ammonia concentrations before and periodically during therapy. Obtain serum levels: Therapeutic serum level range 50–100 mcg/mL.

> **Clinical Tips/Alerts:** May cause *hepatotoxicity*; monitor closely, esp. during initial 6 months of therapy*; fatalities have occurred*. Therapy should be discontinued if hyperammonemia occurs. Life-threatening pancreatitis has also been reported in children and adults. Monitor closely for suicidality in high-risk clients.

Venlafaxine

(ven-la-**fax**-een) Effexor, Effexor XR
Classification: *Therapeutic:* Antidepressants, antianxiety agents; *Pregnancy Category C*
Indications: Major depressive illness or relapse, often in conjunction with psychotherapy. Generalized anxiety disorder (Effexor XR only). Social anxiety disorder (Effexor XR only). **Off-Label Use:** PMDD.
Action: Inhibits serotonin and norepinephrine reuptake in CNS.
Pharmacokinetics: *Absorption:* 92%–100% absorbed after oral administration. *Distribution :* Extensive distribution into body tissues.

DRUGS R-Z

Metabolism and Excretion: Extensively metabolized on first pass through liver. One metabolite, O-desmethylvenlafaxine (ODV), has antidepressant activity; 5% venlafax-ine excreted unchanged in urine; 30% of the active metabolite is excreted in urine.

T ½: *Venlafaxine:* 3–5 hr; *ODV:* 9–11 hr (both ↑ in hepatic/renal impairment).

TIME/ACTION PROFILE (antidepressant action)

Route	Onset	Peak	Duration
PO	Within 2 wk	2–4 wk	Unknown

Contraindicated in: Hypersensitivity; Concurrent MAOI therapy.

Use Cautiously in: CV disease, including hypertension; hepatic impairment (↓ dose recommended); impaired renal function (↓ dose recommended); history of seizures or neurological impairment; history of mania; history of ↑ intraocular pressure or angle-closure glaucoma; observe closely for suicidality and behavior changes; history of drug abuse. **Pregnancy:** Use only if clearly required during pregnancy by weighing benefit to mother versus potential harm to fetus (potential for discontinu-ation syndrome or toxicity in neonate when venlafaxine taken during third trimester). **Lactation:** Potential for serious adverse reactions in infant; discontinue drug or dis-continue breastfeeding.

Adverse Reactions/Side Effects: (CAPITALS indicate life-threatening; underlines indicate most frequent.) **CNS:** SEIZURES, abnormal dreams, anxiety, dizziness, headache, insomnia, nervous-ness, weakness, abnormal thinking, agitation, confusion, depersonalization, drowsi-ness, emotional lability, worsening depression. **EENT:** Rhinitis, visual disturbances, tinnitus. **CV:** Chest pain, hypertension, palpitations, tachycardia. **GI:** Abdominal pain, altered taste, anorexia, constipation, diarrhea, dry mouth, dyspepsia, nausea, vomiting, weight loss. **GU:** Sexual dysfunction, urinary frequency, urinary retention. **Derm:** Ecchymoses, itching, photosensitivity, skin rash. **Neuro:** Paresthesia, twitch-ing. **Misc:** Chills, yawning.

Interactions: Concurrent use with *MAOIs* may result in serious, potentially fatal reac-tions (wait at least 2 wk after stopping MAOI before initiating venlafaxine; wait at least 1 wk after stopping venlafaxine before starting MAOIs). Concurrent use with *alcohol* or other *CNS depressants*, including *sedatives/hypnotics, antihistamines,* and *opioid analgesics,* in depressed clients is not recommended. ↑ Risk of serotonin syn-

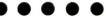

drome with *trazodone, sibutramine, and triptans. Lithium* may have ↑ serotonergic effects with venlafaxine; use cautiously in clients receiving venlafaxine. ↑ Blood levels and may ↑ effects of *desipramine* and *haloperidol. Cimetidine* may ↑ effects of venlafaxine (may be more pronounced in geriatric clients, those with hepatic or renal impairment, and those with pre-existing hypertension). ***Drug-Natural:*** Concomitant use of *kava-kava, valerian, chamomile,* or hops can ↑ CNS depression. ↑ Risk of serotinergic side effects, including serotonin syndrome, with *St. John's wort and SAMe.*

Dosage: PO (Adults): *Tablets:* 75 mg/day in two to three divided doses; may ↑ by up to 75 mg/day every 4 days to 225 mg/day (not to exceed 375 mg/day in three divided doses). *Extended-release (XR) capsules:* 75 mg once daily (some clients may be started at 37.5 mg once daily) for 4–7 days; doses may then be ↑ at intervals of not less than 4 days up to 225 mg/day.

Hepatic Impairment: PO (Adults): ↓ daily dose by 50% in clients with moderate hepatic impairment.

Renal Impairment: PO (Adults): *Mild to moderate renal impairment:* Daily dose should be ↓ by 25%–50%.

Availability (generic available)

Tablets: 25 mg, 37.5 mg, 50 mg, 75 mg, 100 mg. COST: *Generic* **$–$$. Extended-Release Capsules:** 37.5 mg, 75 mg, 150 mg. COST: **$$$$.**

- **Geriatric Considerations:** Caution with CV disease, hypertension, hepatic and renal impairment.
- **Pediatric/Adolescent Considerations:** May be activating; monitor face to face early in treatment for suicidality and during dosage adjustments; ↑ risk for suicidality. May be helpful for anxiety and ADHD. No pediatric indication.
- **Clinical Assessments:** Monitor BP before and during treatment. Sustained hypertension may be dose-related: ↓ Dose or discontinue drug.

Clinical Tips/Alerts: Be aware of dose-related hypertension. Caution with pre-existing hypertension. Less weight gain/sedation and activating for some clients. May be helpful with comorbid anxiety. Do not use concurrently with MAOI (see Interactions).

DRUGS R–Z

Zaleplon

(za-**lep**-lon) Sonata

Classification: Therapeutic: Sedatives/hypnotics; *Schedule IV; Pregnancy Category C*

Indications: Short-term management of insomnia in clients unable to get at least 4 hours of sleep; esp. useful in sleep initiation disorders.

Action: Produces CNS depression by binding to GABA receptors in CNS. Has no analgesic properties.

Pharmacokinetics: *Absorption:* Rapidly absorbed following oral administration.

Distribution: Enters breast milk.

Metabolism and Excretion: Extensively metabolized in liver (mostly by aldehyde oxidase and some by CYP450 3A4 enzymes).

T $1/2$*:* Unknown.

TIME/ACTION PROFILE

Route	Onset	Peak	Duration
PO	Within minutes	Unknown	3–4 hr

Contraindicated in: Hypersensitivity; clients with severe hepatic impairment. *Not recommended for use during pregnancy, lactation.*

Use Cautiously in: Mild to moderate hepatic impairment, age ≥65 yr or weight ≤50 kg or concurrent cimetidine therapy (initiate therapy at lowest dose); impaired respiratory function; history of suicide attempt.

Adverse Reactions/Side Effects: (CAPITALS indicate life-threatening; underlines indicate most frequent.)

CNS: Abnormal thinking, anxiety, behavior changes, depersonalization, dizziness, drowsiness, hallucinations, headache, impaired memory (briefly following dose), impaired psychomotor function (briefly following dose), malaise, sleepdriving, vertigo, weakness. **EENT:** Abnormal vision, ear pain, epistaxis, hearing sensitivity, ocular pain, altered sense of smell. **CV:** Peripheral edema. **GI:** Abdominal pain, anorexia, colitis, dyspepsia, nausea. **GU:** Dysmenorrhea. **Derm:** Photosensitivity. **Neuro:** Hyperesthesia, paresthesia, tremor. **Misc:** Fever, ANAPHYLACTIC REACTION.

Interactions: *Cimetidine* ↑ metabolism and ↑ effects (initiate therapy at a lower dose); Additive CNS depression with other *CNS depressants* including *alcohol, antihistamines, opioid analgesics,* other *sedatives/hypnotics, phenothiazines,* and *tricyclic antidepressants.* Effects may be ↓ by drugs that induce the CYP450 3A4 enzyme system including *rifampin, phenytoin, carbamazepine,* and *phenobarbital.* **Drug-Natural:** Concomitant use of *kava-kava, valerian, chamomile,* or *hops* can ↑ CNS depression. **Drug-Food:** Concurrent ingestion of a *high-fat meal* slows rate of absorption.

Dosage: PO (Adults <65 yr): 10 mg (range 5–20 mg) at bedtime.

PO (Geriatric Clients or Clients <50 kg): Initiate therapy at 5 mg at bedtime (not to exceed 10 mg at bedtime).

Hepatic Impairment: PO (Adults): Initiate therapy at 5 mg at bedtime (not to exceed 10 mg at bedtime).

Availability (generic available)

Capsules: 5 mg, 10 mg. COST: **$**.

- **Geriatric Considerations:** Use cautiously in age ≥65 yr (↓ dose required [5 mg at bedtime]).
- **Pediatric/Adolescent Considerations:** Safety not established for children <18 yr.
- **Substance Abuse Considerations:** Prolonged high-dose prescription (≥7–10 days) may lead to psychological/physical dependence.
- **Clinical Assessments:** Assess sleep patterns before and during treatment.

> **Clinical Tips/Alerts:** Clients have been known to perform activities (cook/eat/drive) *while asleep* (complex sleep-related behaviors) and *serious allergic reactions* have happened (swelling of tongue/throat, difficulty breathing) requiring emergency care. If angioedema develops, seek emergency treatment and do not use drug again. If used for >2 wk, *abrupt withdrawal* may cause dysphoria, insomnia, abdominal or muscle cramps, vomiting, sweating, tremors, and seizures.

Ziprasidone

(zi-**pra**-si-done) Geodon

Classification: *Therapeutic:* Antipsychotics, mood stabilizers; *Pharmacological:* Piperazine derivatives; *Pregnancy Category C*

Indications: Schizophrenia; bipolar mania (manic and manic/mixed episodes). **IM:** Reserved for control of acutely agitated clients.

Action: Effects probably mediated by antagonism of dopamine type 2 (D2) and serotonin type 2 (5-HT$_2$). Also antagonizes alpha$_2$-adrenergic receptors.

Pharmacokinetics: *Absorption:* 60% absorbed following oral administration; 100% absorbed from IM sites.

Distribution: Unknown. Minimal potential for drug interactions due to drug displacement.

Metabolism and Excretion: 99% metabolized by liver; <1% excreted unchanged in urine.

Protein Binding: 99%.

T $\frac{1}{2}$: *PO:* 7 hr; *IM:* 2–5 hr.

TIME/ACTION PROFILE (blood levels)

Route	Onset	Peak	Duration
PO	Within hours	1–3 days*	Unknown
IM	Rapid	60 min	Unknown

*Steady state achieved following continuous use.

Contraindicated in: Hypersensitivity; history of QT prolongation (persistent QTc measurements >500 msec); arrhythmias; recent MI, or uncompensated heart failure; concurrent use of other drugs known to prolong QT interval including quinidine, dofetilide, sotalol, other class Ia and III antiarrhythmics, pimozide, thioridazine, chlorpromazine, droperidol, mefloquine, pentamidine, arsenic trioxide, dolasetron, tacrolimus, droperidol, and moxifloxacin. **Lactation:** Discontinue drug or bottle-feed.

Use Cautiously in: Concurrent diuretic therapy or diarrhea (may ↑ risk of hypotension, hypokalemia, or hypomagnesemia); clients with significant hepatic impairment; history of CV or cerebrovascular disease; hypotension; concurrent antihypertensive therapy, dehydration, or hypovolemia (may ↑ risk of orthostatic hypotension). **Pregnancy:** Use only if potential maternal benefit outweighs potential risk to fetus; geriatric clients (may require ↑ doses; inappropriate use for dementia associated with ↑ mortality); clients at risk for aspiration pneumonia; history of suicide attempt.

Adverse Reactions/Side Effects: (CAPITALS indicate life-threatening; underlines indicate most frequent.)

CNS: NMS, seizures, dizziness, drowsiness, restlessness, extrapyramidal reactions, syncope, tardive dyskinesia. **Resp:** Cough/runny nose. **CV:** PROLONGED QT INTERVAL, orthostatic hypotension. **GI:** Constipation, diarrhea, nausea, dysphagia. **Derm:** Rash, urticaria.

Interactions: Concurrent use of *quinidine, dofetilide, other class Ia and III antiarrhythmics, pimozide, sotalol, thioridazine, chlorpromazine, floquine, pentamidine, arsenic trioxide, mefloquine, dolasetron, tacrolimus, droperidol, moxifloxacin,* or other agents that prolong QT interval may result in potentially life-threatening adverse drug reactions and is contraindicated. Additive CNS depression may occur with *alcohol, antidepressants, antihistamines, opioid analgesics,* or *sedatives/hypnotics.* Blood levels and effectiveness may be ↓ by *carbamazepine.* Blood levels and effects may be ↑ by *ketoconazole.*

Dosage: PO (Adults): *Schizophrenia:* 20 mg twice daily initially; dose increments may be made at 2-day intervals up to 80 mg twice daily. *Acute Mania: Initial Treatment:* 40 mg twice on first day, then 60 or 80 mg twice daily on second day, then 40–80 mg twice daily adjusted based on tolerance and efficacy. *Acute agitation in schizophrenia:* **IM (Adults):** 10–20 mg as needed up to 40 mg/day; may be given as 10 mg every 2 hr or 20 mg every 4 hr.

Availability: Brand only

Capsules: 20 mg, 40 mg, 60 mg, 80 mg. COST: **$$$$. Lyophilized Powder for Injection (Requires Reconstitution):** 20 mg/vial.

- **Geriatric Considerations:** May require reduced dose. ↑ mortality in elderly with dementia-related psychosis.
- **Pediatric/Adolescent Considerations:** Safety not established. Current pediatric studies show efficacy in treatment of bipolar disorder with doses equivalent to those for adults.
- **Clinical Assessments:** ECG before and during prescription; also BP and pulse; weight, BMI, waist circumference, FBS, and lipids before and during prescription. (See *BMI/Metabolic Syndrome, Tools tab.*) Monitor mental status, mood, behaviors, positive and negative symptoms; also EPS, TD, and NMS. (See *Psychotropic Adverse Effects, Basics tab.*)

Clinical Tips/Alerts: Clients found to have persistent QTc measurements of >500 msec should have ziprasidone discontinued. Also see important drug interactions. Monitor for suicidality in high-risk clients. There is no systematic data to guide clinicians in use of ziprasidone in bipolar mania beyond 3 weeks.

Zolpidem

(**zole**-pi-dem) Ambien, Ambien CR

Classification: *Therapeutic:* Sedatives/hypnotics; *Schedule IV; Pregnancy Category B*

Indications: Insomnia.

Action: Produces CNS depression by binding to GABA receptors. Has no analgesic properties.

Pharmacokinetics: *Absorption:* Rapidly absorbed following oral administration. Controlled-release formulation releases 10 mg immediately, then another 2.5 mg later.

Distribution: Minimal amounts enter breast milk; remainder of distribution not known.

Metabolism and Excretion: Converted to inactive metabolites that are excreted by kidneys.

$T_{1/2}$: 2.5–2.6 hr (↑ in geriatric clients and clients with hepatic impairment).

TIME/ACTION PROFILE (sedation)

Route	Onset	Peak*	Duration
PO	Rapid	30 min–2hr	6–8 hr
PO-ER	Rapid	2–4 hr	6–8 hr

*Food delays peak levels and effects.

Contraindicated in: Hypersensitivity; sleep apnea.

Use Cautiously in: History of previous psychiatric illness, suicide attempt, drug or alcohol abuse; clients with pulmonary disease. *Pregnancy or lactation (safety not established).*

Adverse Reactions/Side Effects: (CAPITALS indicate life-threatening; underlines indicate most frequent.)

CNS: Abnormal thinking, amnesia, behavior changes, daytime drowsiness, dizziness, "drugged" feeling, hallucinations, sleep-driving. **GI:** Diarrhea, nausea, vomiting. **Misc:** ANAPHYLACTIC REACTIONS, hypersensitivity reactions, physical dependence, psychological dependence, tolerance.

Interactions: ↑ CNS depression may occur with sedatives/hypnotics, alcohol, phenothiazines, tricyclic antidepressants, opioid analgesics, or antihistamines. *Drug-Natural:* Concomitant use of kava, valerian, or chamomile can ↑ CNS depression. *Drug-Food:* Food ↑ and delays absorption.

Dosage: PO (Adults): *Tablets:* 10 mg at bedtime; *extended-release tablets:* 12.5 mg at bedtime.
PO (Geriatric Clients, Debilitated Clients, or Clients With Hepatic Impairment): *Tablets:* 5 mg at bedtime initially, may be ↑ to 10 mg; *extended-release tablets:* 6.25 mg at bedtime.
Availability (generic available)
Tablets: 5 mg, 10 mg. COST: *Generic* **$. Extended-Release Tablets:** 6.25 mg, 12.5 mg. COST: **$$$**.

- **Geriatric Considerations** Geriatric clients and clients with impaired hepatic function (initial dose reduction recommended [5 mg at bedtime]).
- **Pediatric/Adolescent Considerations:** Safety not established. No current pediatric indications.
- **Substance Abuse Considerations:** Prolonged high-dose treatment (≥7–10 days) may lead to psychological/physical dependence.
- **Clinical Assessments:** Assess sleep patterns before and during treatment.

> **Clinical Tips/Alerts:** Clients have been known to perform activities (cook/eat/drive) *while asleep* (complex sleep-related behaviors) and *serious allergic reactions* have happened (swelling of tongue/throat, difficulty breathing) resulting in emergency care. If angioedema develops, seek emergency treatment and do not use drug again.

Clozaril Protocol: Clozaril Client Management System

Indications for use: Clients with a diagnosis of schizophrenia, unresponsive or intolerant to three different neuroleptics from at least two different therapeutic groups, when given adequate doses for adequate duration.

- System for monitoring white blood cells (WBCs) of clients on clozapine. Important because of possible *(life-threatening) agranulocytosis* and *leukopenia.*
- Need to monitor WBCs, absolute neutrophil count (ANC), and differential before initiating therapy and after.
- WBCs and ANC weekly first 6 mo, then biweekly while Clozaril therapy maintained, then weekly for 1 mo after discontinuation.
- Only available in 1–wk supply (requires WBCs, client monitoring, and controlled distribution through pharmacies).
- If WBC <3000 mm^3 or granulocyte count <1500 mm^3 withhold clozapine (monitor for signs/symptoms of infection).
- Monthly monitoring approved under certain situations (FDA approval 2005).
- Clients must be registered with Clozaril National Registry (see www.clozaril.com).

Common Laboratory Values

General Chemistry

NOTE: Reference ranges vary according to brand of laboratory assay materials used. Check normal reference ranges from your facility's laboratory when evaluating results.

Lab	Conventional	SI Units
Albumin	3.5–5 g/100 mL	35–50 g/L
Aldolase	1.3–8.2 U/L	22–137 nmol sec^{-1}/L
Alkaline phosphatase	13–39 U/L; infants and adolescents up to 104 U/L	217–650 nmol sec^{-1}/L up to 1.26 μmol/L
Ammonia	12–55 μmol/L	12–55 μmol/L
Amylase	4–25 unit/mL	4–25 arb unit

Lab	Conventional	SI Units
Anion gap	8–16 mEq/L	8–16 mmol/L
ALT	10–35 U/L	0–58 μkat/L
AST	0–35 U/L	0–0.58 μkat/L
Bilirubin, direct	Up to 0.4 mg/100 mL	Up to 7 μmol/L
Bilirubin, total	Up to 1 mg/100 mL	Up to 17 μmol/L
Blood urea nitrogen	8–25 mg/100 mL	2.9–8.9 mmol/L
Calcitonin	Male: 0–14 pg/mL	0–4.1 pmol/L
	Female: 0–28 pg/mL	0–8.2 pmol/L
Calcium	8.5–10.5 mg/100 mL	2.1–2.6 mmol/L
Carbon dioxide	24–30 mEq/L	24–30 mmol/L
Chloride	100–106 mEq/L	100–106 mmol/L
Cholesterol	<200 mg/dL	<5.18 mmol/L
Cortisol	(a.m.) 5–25 mcg/100 mL	0.14–0.69 μmol/L
	(p.m.) <10 μg/100 mL	0–0.28 μmol/L
Creatine	Male: 0.2–0.5 mg/dL	15–40 μmol/L
	Female: 0.3–0.9 mg/dL	25–70 μmol/L
Creatine kinase	Male: 17–148 U/L	283–2467 nmol sec^{-1}/L
	Female: 10–79 U/L	167–1317 nmol sec^{-1}/L
Creatinine	0.6–1.5 mg/100 mL	53–133 μmol/L
Ferritin	10–410 ng/dL	10–410 mcg/dL
Folate	2–9 ng/mL	4.5–20.4 nmol/L
Glucose	70–110 mg/100 mL	3.9–5.6 mmol/L
Ionized calcium	4.25–5.25 mg/dL	1.1–1.3 mmol/L
Iron	50–150 mcg/100 mL	9–26.9 μmol/L
Iron-binding capacity	250–410 mcg/100 mL	44.8–73.4 μmol/L
Lactic acid	0.6–1.8 mEq/L	0.6–1.8 mmol/L
Lactic dehydrogenase	45–90 U/L	750–1500 nmol sec^{-1}/L
Lipase	2 units/mL or less	Up to 2 arb unit

Lab	Conventional	SI Units
Magnesium	1.5–2 mEq/L	0.8–1.3 mmol/L
Osmolality	280–296 mOsm/kg water	280–296 mmol/kg
Phosphorus	3–4.5 mg/100 mL	1–1.5 mmol/L
Potassium	3.5–5 mEq/L	3.5–5 mmol/L
Prealbumin	18–32 mg/dL	180–320 mg/L
Prostate-specific antigen	<4 ng/mL	<4 µg/L
Protein, total	6–8.4 g/100 mL	60–84 g/L
Pyruvate	0–0.11 mEq/L	0–0.11 mmol/L
Sodium	135–145 mEq/L	135–145 mmol/L
T3	75–195 ng/100 mL	1.16–3 nmol/L
T4, free	Male: 0.8—1.8 ng/dL	10–23 pmol/L
	Female: 0.8—1.8 ng/dL	10–23 pmol/L
T4, total	4–12 mcg/100 mL	52–154 nmol/L
Thyroglobulin	3–42 ng/mL	3–42 µg/L
Thyroid-stimulating hormone	0.4–4.2 µIU/mL	0.4–4.2 mU/L
Triglycerides	40–150 mg/100 mL	0.4–1.5 g/L
Urea nitrogen	8–25 mg/100 mL	2.9–8.9 mmol/L
Uric acid	3–7 mg/100 mL	0.18–0.42 mmol/L

Hematology

Lab	Conventional	SI Units
Blood volume	8.5%–9% of body weight in kg	80–85 mL/kg
Red blood cells	Male: 4.6–6.2 million/mm³; Female: 4.2–5.9 million/mm³	4.6–6.2 × 10^{12}/L; 4.2–5.9 × 10^{12}/L
Hemoglobin	Male: 13–18 g/100 mL; Female: 12–16 g/100 mL	Male: 8.1–11.2 mmol/L; Female: 7.4–9.9 mmol/L

Lab	Conventional	SI Units
Hematocrit	Male: 45%–52%	Male: 0.45–0.52
	Female: 37%–48%	Female: 0.37–0.48
Leukocytes (WBCs)	4300–10,800/mm^3	4.3–10.8 × 10^9/L
• Bands	0%–5%	0.03–0.08 × 10^9/L
• Basophils	0%–1%	0–0.01 × 10^9/L
• Eosinophils	1%–4%	0.01–0.04 × 10^9/L
• Lymphocytes	25%–40%	0.25–0.40 × 10^9/L
• B-lymphocytes	10%–20%	0.10–0.20 × 10^9/L
• T-lymphocytes	60%–80%	0.60–0.80 × 10^9/L
• Monocytes	2%–8%	0.02–0.08 × 10^9/L
• Neutrophils	54%–75%	0.54–0.75 × 10^9/L
Platelets	150,000–350,000/mm^3	150–350 × 10^9/L
Erythrocyte sedimentation rate	Male: 1–13 mm/hr	Male: 1–13 mm/hr
	Female: 1–20 mm/hr	Female: 1–20 mm/hr

Treatment Algorithms in Psychopharmacology

Psychiatric algorithms have been devised to assist in the psychotropic treatment decision-making process (Fawcett J, Stein DJ, Jobson KO, 1999). Extensive work and research on treatment algorithms continue to be done by the International Psychopharmacology Algorithm Project (IPAP) (www.ipap.org).

Important: All IPAP algorithms are of a general and theoretical nature and are for educational and instructive purposes only for health professionals and researchers and are not for prescriptive use.

Go to *DavisPlus* (http://davisplus.fadavis.com) for the following IPAP algorithms under General Resources: Generalized Anxiety Disorder Algorithm (English and Spanish), Post-Traumatic Stress Disorder Algorithm (English and Spanish), and Schizophrenia Algorithm.

Following is an **IPAP algorithm for schizophrenia:**

**LABS/
PROTOCOLS**

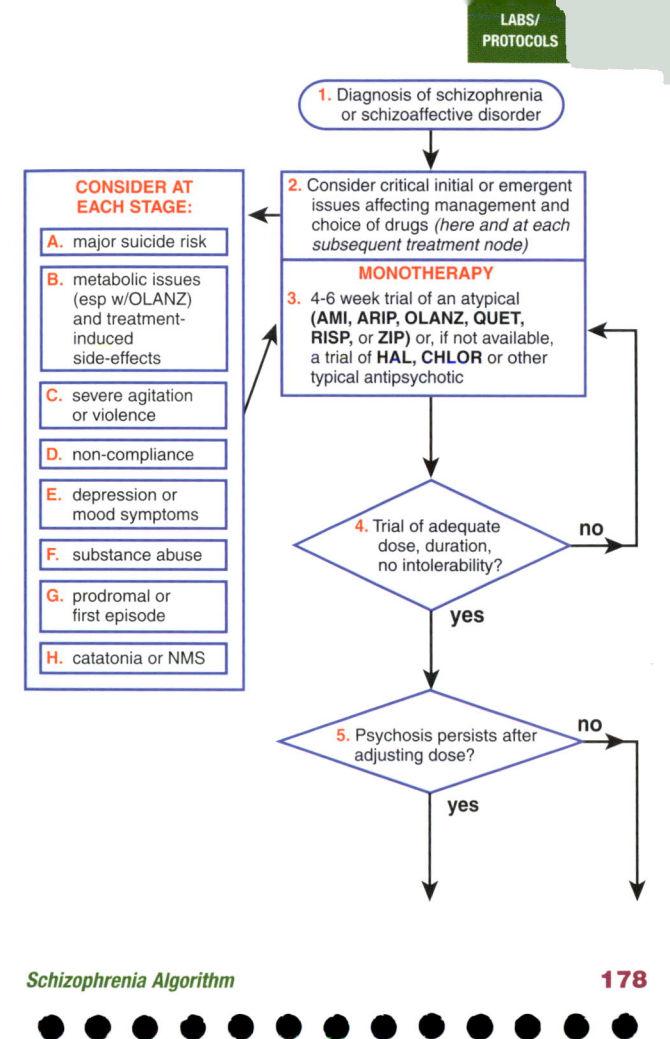

1. Diagnosis of schizophrenia or schizoaffective disorder

2. Consider critical initial or emergent issues affecting management and choice of drugs *(here and at each subsequent treatment node)*

CONSIDER AT EACH STAGE:

A. major suicide risk

B. metabolic issues (esp w/OLANZ) and treatment-induced side-effects

C. severe agitation or violence

D. non-compliance

E. depression or mood symptoms

F. substance abuse

G. prodromal or first episode

H. catatonia or NMS

MONOTHERAPY

3. 4-6 week trial of an atypical **(AMI, ARIP, OLANZ, QUET, RISP,** or **ZIP)** or, if not available, a trial of **HAL, CHLOR** or other typical antipsychotic

4. Trial of adequate dose, duration, no intolerability?   **no**

yes

5. Psychosis persists after adjusting dose?   **no**

yes

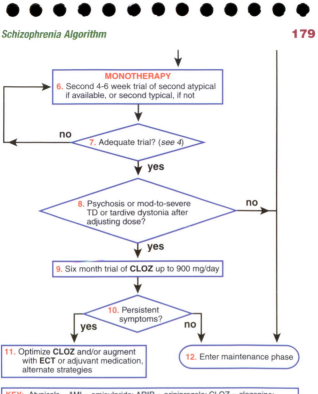

MONOTHERAPY

6. Second 4-6 week trial of second atypical if available, or second typical, if not

7. Adequate trial? (*see 4*) — **no**

yes

8. Psychosis or mod-to-severe TD or tardive dystonia after adjusting dose? — **no**

yes

9. Six month trial of **CLOZ** up to 900 mg/day

10. Persistent symptoms?

yes   **no**

11. Optimize **CLOZ** and/or augment with **ECT** or adjuvant medication, alternate strategies

12. Enter maintenance phase

KEY: Atypicals – AMI = amisulpride; ARIP = aripiprazole; CLOZ = clozapine; OLANZ = olanzapine; QUET = quetiapine; RISP = risperidone; ZIP = ziprasidone. Typicals — CHLOR = chlorpromazine; FLU = fluphenazine; HAL = haloperidol; THIO = thiothixene. Other — AD = antidepressant; BZD = benzodiazepine; ECT = electroconvulsive therapy; IM = intramuscular; MS = mood stabilizer; TD = tardive dyskinesia; NMS = Neuroleptic Malignant Syndrome

IPAP Schizophrenia Algorithm. Copyright 2004–2006. International Psychopharmacology Algorithm Project (IPAP) www.ipap.org

LABS/ PROTOCOLS

Tools

Go to DavisPlus

(http://davisplus.fadavis.com) **for the following:**

- Animations for anxiety, depression, schizophrenia, and pharmacokinetics (ADME)
- Client education teaching guidelines (client/family handouts)
- Davis' dosage calculator
- IPAP algorithms (schizophrenia, GAD, PTSD)
- Laboratory medication levels (antidepressants, antipsychotics, antimanics)
- Medication Assessment Tool
- Preventing medication errors
- Psychotropic drug monographs, including SAMe and St. John's wort
- Psychotropic medication tutorial
- Syringe compatibility chart; syringe exercises

Trade Names to Generic Names (Drugs A-Z)*

- Abilify—aripiprazole
- Adderall—amphetamine mixtures
- Ambien—zolpidem
- Anafranil—clomipramine
- Aricept—donepezil
- Artane—trihexyphenidyl
- Atarax—hydroxyzine
- Ativan—lorazepam
- BuSpar—buspirone
- Celexa—citalopram
- Catapres—clonidine
- Clozaril—clozapine
- Cogentin—benztropine
- Cognex—tacrine
- Concerta—methylphenidate
- Cymbalta—duloxetine
- Dalmane—flurazepam
- Daytrana—methylphenidate transdermal
- Depakote—valproates

- Desyrel—trazodone
- Dexedrine—dextroamphetamine
- Effexor—venlafaxine
- Elavil—amitriptyline
- Emsam—selegiline transdermal
- Exelon—rivastigmine
- Geodon—ziprasidone
- Halcion—triazolam
- Haldol—haloperidol
- Inderal—propranolol
- Invega—paliperidone
- Klonopin—clonazepam
- Lamictal—lamotrigine
- Lexapro—escitalopram
- Librium—chlordiazepoxide
- Lithobid—lithium
- Loxitane—loxapine
- Luminal—phenobarbital
- Lunesta—eszopiclone
- Luvox—fluvoxamine
- Marplan—isocarboxazid
- Mellaril—thioridazine
- Moban—molindone
- Namenda—memantine
- Nardil—phenelzine
- Navane—thiothixene
- Neurontin—gabapentin
- Norpramin—desipramine
- Orap—pimozide
- Pamelor—nortriptyline
- Parnate—tranylcypromine
- Paxil—paroxetine hydrochloride
- Pristiq—desvenlafaxine
- Prolixin—fluphenazine
- Prozac—fluoxetine
- Razadyne—galantamine

- Remeron—mirtazapine
- Restoril—temazepam
- Risperdal—risperidone
- Ritalin—methylphenidate
- Rozerem—ramelteon
- Serax—oxazepam
- Seroquel—quetiapine
- Serzone—nefazodone
- Sinequan—doxepin
- Sonata—zaleplon
- Strattera—atomoxetine
- Symbyax—olanzapine and fluoxetine
- Tegretol—carbamazepine
- Thorazine—chlorpromazine
- Tofranil—imipramine
- Topamax—topiramate
- Trilafon—perphenazine
- Valium—diazepam
- Wellbutrin—bupropion
- Xanax—alprazolam
- Zoloft—sertraline
- Zyprexa—olanzapine

*The preceding trade names are only examples of one common trade name for each generic drug. These do not include all possible trade names nor do they intend to suggest that any specific trade drug be used in place of another. This is meant to serve as a helpful tool in locating a generic drug equivalent within the alphabetical drug listing.

Abbreviations

ABG—arterial blood gas
ac—before meals
AD—dementia of Alzheimer's type
ADHD—attention deficit–hyperactivity disorder
AIMS—Abnormal Involuntary Movement Scale

BID—twice daily
BMI—body mass index
BP—blood pressure
BPH—benign prostatic hypertrophy
BUN—blood urea nitrogen
cap—capsule
CBC—complete blood count
CBT—cognitive behavioral therapy
CCr—creatinine clearance
CHF—congestive heart failure
CK—creatinine kinase
CNS—central nervous system
COPD—chronic obstructive pulmonary disease
CPK—creatine phosphokinase
CR—controlled-release
CV—cardiovascular
derm—dermatologic
dL—deciliter
ECG—electrocardiogram
ECT—electroconvulsive therapy
EENT—eye, ear, nose, and throat
endo—endocrine
EPS—extrapyramidal symptoms
ER—extended-release
ESRD—end-stage renal disease
F&E—fluid and electrolyte
FBS—fasting blood sugar
g—gram
GABA—gamma-aminobutyric acid
GAD—generalized anxiety disorder
GERD—gastroesophageal reflux disease
GFR—glomerular filtration rate
GI—gastrointestinal
GTT—glucose tolerance test
GU—genitourinary
HDL—high-density lipoproteins

hemat—hematological
HF—heart failure
Hgb A1C—hemoglobin A1c, glycosylated hemoglobin (blood sugar averages)
hr—hour
IBS—irritable bowel syndrome
IM—intramuscular
inhaln—inhalation
IV—intravenous
K—potassium
KCl—potassium chloride
kg—kilogram
L—liter
LA—long-acting
LDH—lactic dehydrogenase
LDL—low-density lipoproteins
LFT—liver function test
M—molar
MAOI—monoamine oxidase inhibitor
mcg—microgram
MDD—major depressive disorder
mEq—milliequivalent
metab—metabolic
mg—milligram
min—minute
misc—miscellaneous
mL—milliliter
mM—millimole
MRI—magnetic resonance imaging
MS—musculoskeletal
Na—sodium
NaCl—sodium chloride
NE—norepinephrine
neuro—neurological
NMS—neuroleptic malignant syndrome
NPO—nothing by mouth

NSAID—nonsteroidal anti-inflammatory drug
OCD—obsessive-compulsive disorder
ophth—ophthalmic
OTC—over-the-counter
pc—after meals
PMDD—premenstrual dysphoric disorder
PO—by mouth, orally
prn—as needed
PT—prothrombin time
PTT—partial thromboplastin time
PVC—premature ventricular contraction
RBC—red blood cell
rect—rectally or rectal
resp—respiratory
Rx—prescription
sec—second
SL—sublingual
SNRI—serotonin-norepinephrine reuptake inhibitor
SR—sustained-release
SSRI—selective serotonin reuptake inhibitor
stat—immediately
subcut—subcutaneous
supp—suppository
T$^{1}/_{2}$—half life
tab—tablet
tbs—tablespoon
TFT—thyroid function test
top—topically or topical
tsp—teaspoon
UA—urinalysis
UK—unknown
UTI—urinary tract infection
VLDL—very low–density lipoproteins
WBC—white blood cell
wk—week
yr—year

Psychotropic Approximate Dose Equivalences*

● **Benzodiazepines:**
- Ativan (lorazepam) — 1 mg
- Klonopin (clonazepam) — 0.5 mg
- Librium (chlordiazepoxate) — 10 mg
- Serax (oxazepam) — 15 mg
- Tranxene (clorazepate) — 7.5 mg
- Valium (diazepam) — 5 mg
- Xanax/Xanax XR (alprazolam/ER) — 0.5 mg

● **Psychostimulants:**
- Adderall (amphetamine salts) — 7.5 mg BID
- Adderall XR (amphetamine salts XR) — 15 mg
- Concerta (methylphenidate ER) — 18 mg
- Daytrana (methylphenidate transdermal) — 20 mg
- Dexedrine (dextroamphetamine) — 15 mg
- Focalin (dexmethylphenidate) — 5 mg BID
- Focalin XR (dexmethylphenidate ER) — 10 mg
- Metadate ER/CD (methylphenidate ER) — 15 mg
- Ritalin (methylphenidate) — 5 mg TID
- Ritalin SR/LA (methylphenidate ER) — 15 mg
- Vyvanse (lisdexamfetamine) — 20–30 mg

● **Serotonin Reuptake Inhibitor Antidepressants:**
- Celexa (citalopram) — 20 mg
- Lexapro (escitalopram) — 10 mg
- Luvox (fluvoxamine) — 50 mg BID
- Luvox CR (fluvoxamine ER) — 100 mg
- Paxil (paroxetine) — 20 mg
- Paxil CR (paroxetine CR) — 25 mg
- Prozac/Serafem (fluoxetine) — 20 mg
- Prozac Weekly (fluoxetine wkly) — 90 mg/wk
- Zoloft (sertraline) — 50 mg

● **Atypicals (2nd/3rd Generation) Antipsychotics:**
- Abilify (aripiprazole) — 15 mg
- Geodon (ziprasidone) — 40 mg BID
- Invega (paliperidone) — 6 mg

- Risperdal (risperidone)   1 mg BID
- Seroquel (quetiapine)   100 mg BID
- Seroquel XR (quetiapine ER)   200 mg
- Zyprexa (olanzepine)   10 mg

Typicals (1st Generation) Antipsychotics:
- Haldol (haloperidol)   2 mg
- Loxitane (loxapine)   10 mg
- Mellaril (thioridazine)   100 mg
- Moban (molindone)   10 mg
- Navane (thiothixene)   5 mg
- Prolixin (fluphenazine)   2 mg
- Thorazine (chlorpromazine)   100 mg
- Trilafon (perphenazine)   16 mg

Nonbenzodiazepine Hypnotics & Sleep Aids:
- Ambien (zolpidem)   10 mg
- Ambien CR (zolpidem ER)   12.5 mg
- Benadryl (diphenhydramine)   25–50 mg
- Buspar (buspirone)   10 mg
- Desyrel (trazodone)   50–100 mg
- Lunesta (eszopiclone)   3 mg
- Rozerem (ramelteon)   8 mg
- Sonata (zaleplon)   10 mg
- Vistaril (hydroxyzine)   50 mg

Benzodiazepine Hypnotics & Sleep Aids:
- Dalmane (flurazepan)   15–30 mg
- Doral (quazepam)   20 mg
- Halcion (triazolam)   0.5 mg
- ProSom (estazolam)   1–2 mg
- Restoril (temazepam)   15 mg

*ALERT: The Psychotropic Approximate Dose Equivalences are intended as guide-lines only. See the drug alert on the inside front cover, which applies to these dose equivalences as well as all drugs.

TOOLS/ INDEX

Pregnancy Categories and Controlled Substances Schedules

PREGNANCY CATEGORIES

Category A

Adequate, well-controlled studies in pregnant women have not shown an increased risk of fetal abnormalities.

Category B

Animal studies have revealed no evidence of harm to the fetus; however, there are no adequate and well-controlled studies in pregnant women. OR Animal studies have shown an adverse effect, but adequate and well-controlled studies in pregnant women have failed to demonstrate a risk to the fetus.

Category C

Animal studies have shown an adverse effect, and there are no adequate and well-controlled studies in pregnant women. OR No animal studies have been conducted, and there are no adequate and well-controlled studies in pregnant women.

Category D

Studies, adequate or well-controlled, in pregnant women have demonstrated a risk to the fetus. However, the benefits of therapy may outweigh the potential risk.

Category X

Studies, adequate and well-controlled or observational, in animals or pregnant women have demonstrated positive evidence of fetal abnormalities. The use of the product is contraindicated in women who are or may become pregnant.

NOTE: The designation UK is used when the pregnancy category is unknown.

CONTROLLED SUBSTANCES SCHEDULES

Classes or schedules are determined by the Drug Enforcement Agency (DEA), an arm of the United States Justice Department, and are based on the potential for abuse and dependence liability (physical and psychological) of the medication. Some states may have stricter prescription regulations. Physicians, dentists, podiatrists, and veterinarians may prescribe controlled substances. Nurse practitioners and physician assistants may prescribe controlled substances with certain limitations.

Schedule I (C-I)

Potential for abuse is so high as to be unacceptable. May be used for research with appropriate limitations. Examples are LSD and heroin.

Schedule II (C-II)

High potential for abuse and extreme liability for physical and psychological dependence (amphetamines, opioid analgesics, dronabinol, certain barbiturates). Outpatient prescriptions must be in writing. In emergencies, telephone orders may be acceptable if a written prescription is provided within 72 hours. No refills are allowed. Pharmacy must receive an original hard-copy prescription or triplicate for each supply.

Schedule III (C-III)

Intermediate potential for abuse (less than C-II) and intermediate liability for physical and psychological dependence (certain nonbarbiturate sedatives, certain nonamphetamine CNS stimulants, and certain opioid analgesics). Outpatient prescriptions can be refilled five times within 6 months from date of issue if authorized by prescriber. Telephone orders are acceptable.

Schedule IV (C-IV)

Less abuse potential than Schedule III with minimal liability for physical or psychological dependence (certain sedative/hypnotics, certain antianxiety agents, some barbiturates, benzodiazepines, chloral hydrate, pentazocine, and propoxyphene). Outpatient prescriptions can be refilled 6 times within 6 months from date of issue if authorized by prescriber. Telephone orders are acceptable.

Schedule V (C-V)

Minimal abuse potential. Number of outpatient refills determined by prescriber. Some products (cough suppressants with small amounts of codeine, antidiarrheals)

BMI/Metabolic Syndrome

BMI Chart (English and Metric)

The intersection of your weight and height equals your BMI. A BMI greater than 30 puts client at greatest risk for cardiovascular disease/diabetes and other disorders. Risk increases between 25 to 29 and the preferred BMI is between 19 and 24. A BMI of <18 is considered underweight. (National Institutes of Health: Clinical Guidelines on the Identification, Evaluation, and Treatment of Overweight and Obesity in Adults: The Evidence Report, September 1998)

(Lutz & Przytulski, NutriNotes, Philadelphia: FA Davis, 2004, used with permission.)

TOOLS/ INDEX

TOOLS/INDEX

Body Mass Index Chart (English and Metric)

Body Mass Index (BMI) is an indicator of optimal weight for health. Find the intersection of your weight and height—this is your BMI. Adults with a BMI between 19 and 24 have less risk for illnesses such as heart disease and diabetes than individuals with a BMI between 25 and 29. A BMI greater than 30 indicates greatest risk for obesity-related diseases. Adapted from the National Institute of Health, NHLBI Clinical Guidelines on Overweight and Obesity, June 1988, www.nhlbi.nih.gov/guidelines

Legend: ☐ Underweight ☐ Weight Appropriate ☐ Overweight ☐ Obese

Height (feet and inches): 5'0", 5'1", 5'2", 5'3", 5'4", 5'5", 5'6", 5'7", 5'8", 5'9", 5'10", 5'11", 6'0"

Weight (lb)	150	152.5	155	157.5	160	162.5	165	167.5	170	172.5	175	177.5	180	Weight (kg)
100	20	19	18	18	17	17	16	16	15	15	14	14	14	45
105	21	20	19	19	18	17	17	16	16	16	15	15	14	47
110	21	21	20	19	19	18	18	17	17	16	16	15	15	50
115	22	22	21	20	20	19	19	18	17	17	17	16	16	52
120	23	23	22	21	21	20	19	19	18	18	17	17	16	54
125	24	24	23	22	21	21	20	20	19	18	18	17	17	57
130	25	25	24	23	22	22	21	20	20	19	19	18	18	59
135	26	26	25	24	23	22	22	21	21	20	19	19	18	61
140	27	26	26	25	24	23	23	22	21	21	20	20	19	63
145	28	27	27	26	25	24	23	23	22	21	21	20	20	66
150	29	28	27	27	26	25	24	23	23	22	22	21	20	68
155	30	29	28	27	27	26	25	24	24	23	22	22	21	70
160	31	30	29	28	27	27	26	25	24	24	23	22	22	73
165	32	31	30	29	28	27	27	26	25	24	24	23	22	75
170	33	32	31	30	29	28	27	27	26	25	24	24	23	77
175	34	33	32	31	30	29	28	27	27	26	25	24	24	79
180	35	34	33	32	31	30	29	28	27	27	26	25	24	82
185	36	35	34	33	32	31	30	29	28	27	27	26	25	84
190	37	36	35	34	33	32	31	30	29	28	27	27	26	86
195	38	37	36	35	33	32	31	31	30	29	28	27	26	88
200	39	38	37	35	34	33	32	31	30	30	29	28	27	91
205	40	39	37	36	35	34	33	32	31	30	29	29	28	93
210	41	40	38	37	36	35	34	33	32	31	30	29	28	96
215	42	41	39	38	37	36	35	34	33	32	31	30	29	98
220	43	42	40	39	38	37	36	34	33	32	32	31	30	100
225	44	43	41	40	39	37	36	35	34	33	32	31	31	102
230	45	43	42	41	39	38	37	36	35	34	33	32	31	104
235	46	44	43	42	40	39	38	37	36	35	34	33	32	107
240	47	45	44	43	41	40	39	38	36	35	34	33	33	109
245	47	46	45	43	42	41	40	38	37	36	35	34	33	111
250	49	47	46	44	43	42	40	39	38	37	36	35	34	114

Height (centimeters)

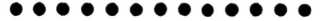

Metabolic Syndrome

Metabolic syndrome is defined as a group of clinical symptoms/criteria including abdominal obesity, hypertension, and diabetes as well as low high-density lipoprotein levels and high levels of triglycerides. There is now a greater concern about the development of metabolic syndrome for those prescribed antipsychotics (Remington 2006). It is important to monitor waist circumference, BMI, weight, blood pressure, lipids, fasting blood sugar, and HgB A1c, if diabetic.

Waist circumference should be <40 inches (102 cm) for men and <35 inches (88 cm) for women.

Clinical Identification of Metabolic Syndrome

Any three of the following:

Risk Factor	Defining Level
Abdominal Obesity	*Waist Circumference*
Men	>102 cm (>40 in)
Women	>88 cm (>35 in)
Triglycerides	>150 mg/dL
HDL cholesterol	
Men	<40 mg/dL
Women	<50 mg/dL
Blood pressure	>130/>85 mm Hg
Fasting glucose	>110 mg/dL

National Institutes of Health. ATP III Guidelines (National Cholesterol Education Program), NIH Publication No. 01-3305.

MAOI Diet (Tyramine) Restrictions

FOODS: MUST AVOID COMPLETELY

- Aged red wines (cabernet sauvignon/merlot/chianti)
- Aged (smoked, pickled, fermented, marinated, and processed) meats (pepperoni/bologna/salami, pickled herring, liver, frankfurters, bacon, ham)

● Aged/mature cheeses (blue/cheddar/provolone/brie/romano/parmesan/ swiss)
● Overripe fruits and vegetables (overripe bananas/sauerkraut/all overripe fruit)
● Beans (fava, Italian, Chinese pea pod, fermented bean curd, soya sauce, tofu, miso soup)
● Condiments (bouillon cubes/meat tenderizers/canned soups/gravy/sauces/soy sauce)
● Soups (prepared/canned/frozen)
● Beverages (beer/ales/vermouth/whiskey/liqueurs/nonalcoholic wines and beers)

FOODS: USE WITH CAUTION (moderation)

● Avocados (not overripe)
● Raspberries (small amounts)
● Chocolate (small amount)
● Caffeine (2–8-oz. servings per day or less)
● Dairy products (limit to buttermilk, yogurt, sour cream [small amounts], cream cheese, cottage cheese, milk if fresh)

MEDICATIONS: MUST AVOID

● Stimulants
● Decongestants
● OTC medications (check with practitioner (MD or APN)/pharmacist)
● Opioids
● Meperidine
● Ephedrine/epinephrine
● Methyldopa
● Herbal remedies

Any questions about foods, OTC medications, herbals, and medications (newly prescribed) should be discussed with the psychiatrist, pharmacist, or advanced practice nurse because of serious nature of any food-drug, drug-drug combinations.

Nonpharmacological Treatments of Depression/Other Disorders

Although pharmacological treatments provide often necessary and appropriate treatment of psychiatric disorders, there are other nonpharmacological treatments that may be used in conjunction with or in some instances instead of prescribed psychotropics. It is important to keep abreast of both novel and other approved treatments for a well-rounded treatment armamentarium (Botai, 2008).

Transcranial Magnetic Stimulation

Noninvasive technique to treat brain physiology that produces repetitive electrical currents to the brain to treat major depression, auditory hallucinations, and other neurological disorders (migraine, Parkinson's). Has been shown to have antidepressant effects (Stern et al, 2007); more studies are needed to demonstrate long-term effectiveness.

Vagal Nerve Stimulation

Adjunctive long-term treatment of chronic depression (not responsive to four or more adequate antidepressant treatments) that uses a small implantable device (Cyberonics Inc., 2005; Fitzgerald & Daskalakis, 2008)

Cognitive Behavioral Therapy (CBT)

CBT is a proven nonpharmalogical treatment of depression and anxiety disorders (panic, GAD, phobias, OCD). It is often very effective when used in conjunction with psychopharmacology (e.g., fluoxetine and CBT for OCD) (Freeman et al., 2004).

Natural/Herbal Products

Natural products such as St. John's wort and SAMe may help with depression when symptoms are mild/possibly moderate. These products are discussed in the alphabetical drug tab. They should not be combined with other antidepressants but used instead of prescribed antidepressants if they are effective.

Other Complementary Therapies

Therapies that may complement pharmacological treatments include light therapy, meditation, biofeedback, art therapy, prayer, acupressure, acupuncture, humor therapy, and pet therapy, to name a few. These therapies should complement traditional treatments and can be very effective in the treatment of pain, stress, insomnia, depression, and other symptoms/disorders.

References

Ahuja N, Palanichamy N, Mackin P, et al. Olanzapine-induced hyperglycaemic coma and neuroleptic malignant syndrome: Case report and review of literature. J Psychopharmacol Sep 18, 2008.

Botai T. Non-drug treatment for depression. Presse Med 37(5 Pt 2):877–882, 2008.

Cyberonics Inc., 2007. Vagal nerve stimulation. Accessed 9/27/08 at www.vnstherapy.com

Deglin JH, Vallerand AH: Davis's drug guide for nurses, ed 11. FA Davis, Philadelphia, 2009.

Evans DL, Foa EB, Gur RE, et al. Treating and preventing adolescent mental health disorders: A research agenda. Oxford University Press, Oxford/New York, 2005.

Fawcett J, Stein DJ, Jobson KO. Textbook of treatment algorithms in psychopharmacology, Wiley, New York, 1999.

FDA: Center for Drug Evaluation and Research. Accessed for drug information and black box warnings at www.fda.gov/cder/index

Fitzgerald PB, Daskalakis ZJ. The use of repetitive transcranial magnetic stimulation and vagal nerve stimulation in the treatment of depression. Curr Opin Psychiatry 21:25-29, 2008.

Fuller MA: Drug information handbook for psychiatry: A comprehensive reference of psychotropic, nonpsychotropic, and herbal agents, ed 6. Lexi-Comp, Cleveland, 2007.

Jones LD, Payne ME, Messer DF, et al. Temporal lobe volume in bipolar disorder: Relationship with diagnosis and antipsychotic medication use. J Affect Discord Aug 6, 2008.

Krishnan KR. Psychiatric and medical comorbidities of bipolar disorder. Psychosomatic Med 67:1-8, 2005.

Martin A, Bostic JQ. Psychopharmacology. Child Adolesc Psychiatric Clin North Am 15:1, 2006.

Maxman JS, Ward NG. Psychotropic drugs fast facts, ed 3. WW Norton, New York, 2002.

Meador KJ, et al. Cognitive function at 3 years of age after fetal exposure to antiepileptic drugs. N Engl J Med 360(16): 1597-1605, 2009.

Meador KJ, et al. In utero antiepileptic drug exposure: Fetal death and malformations. Neurology 67(3):407-412, 2006.

Remington G. Schizophrenia, antipsychotics, and the metabolic syndrome: Is there a silver lining? [editorial] Am J Psychiatry 163:7, 2006.

National Institutes of Health. ATP III Guidelines (National Cholesterol Education Program). NIH Publication No. 01-3305, May 2001.

National Institutes of Health. Clinical guidelines on the identification, evaluation, and treatment of overweight and obesity in adults: The evidence report (Obesity Education Initiative). NIH Publication No. 98-4083, September 1998

Pedersen D. PsychNotes: Clinical pocket guide, ed 2. FA Davis, Philadelphia, 2008.

Rosenbaum JF, Arana GW, Hyman SE, et al. Handbook of psychiatric drug therapy, ed 5. Lippincott Williams & Wilkins, Philadelphia, 2005.

Stern WM, Tormos JM, Press DZ, et al. Antidepressant effects of high- and low-frequency repetitive transcranial magnetic stimulation to the dorsolateral prefrontal cortex: A double-blind, randomized, placebo-controlled trial. J Neuropsychiatry Clin Neurosci 19:179-186, 2007.

Taylor WD, Doraiswamy PM, Krishnan KR. Evidence-based treatment of psychiatric disorders with comorbid medical illnesses: The need for large simple clinical trials. Pyschopharmacol Bull 40:5-11, 2007.

Townsend MC. Psychiatric mental health nursing: Concepts of care in evidence-based practice, ed 6. FA Davis, Philadelphia, 2009.

US Food and Drug Administration: FDA is requiring the manufacturers of conventional antipsychotic drugs to add a *Boxed Warning* and *Warning* to the drugs' prescribing information about the risk of mortality in elderly patients treated for dementia-related psychosis. Accessed 9/27/2008 at www.fda.gov/CDER/drug/InfoSheets/HCP/antipsychotics_conventional.htm

Credits:

Content, including dosages and drug data (indications, adverse reactions, interactions, etc.), psychotropic medication tutorial, syringe compatibility chart, dosage calculator, and preventing medication errors have been used from the following with permission of the Publisher: Deglin JH, Vallerand AH: Davis's drug guide for nurses, ed 11, FA Davis, Philadelpia, 2009.

Laboratory data (general chemistry, hematology) have been used with permission from Myers E. RNotes, ed 2. Philadelphia: FA Davis, 2006 and also Hopkins, Lab Notes, 2005.

Also used with permission are animations and client teaching guides from Townsend 2009 to be used on DavisPlus, as well as lab medication levels (on DavisPlus and in text) from Van Leeuwen et al: Davis's comprehensive handbook of laboratory and diagnostic tests with nursing implications, 2e, 2006; and from Castillo et al: Calculating drug dosages, 2e, 2007, syringe exercises.

TOOLS/INDEX

Index